Healthy, Natural Estrogens f

Copyright © 2013 by Susan M. Lark, M.D.

All rights reserved. No part of this book may be reproduced or transmitted in any form or by any means, electronic or mechanical, including photocopying, recording, or by any information storage or retrieval system, without permission in writing from the Publisher.

Womens Wellness Publishing, LLC
www.womenswellnesspublishing.com
www.facebook.com/wwpublishing

Mention of specific companies or products in this book does not suggest endorsement by the author or publisher. Internet addresses and telephone numbers for resources provided in this book were accurate at the time it went to press.

Cover design by Rebecca Rose

ISBN 978-1-939013-85-9

Note: The information in this book is meant to complement the advice and guidance of your physician, not replace it. It is very important that women who have medical problems be evaluated by a physician. If you are under the care of a physician, you should discuss any major changes in your regimen with him or her. Because this is a book and not a medical consultation, keep in mind that the information presented here may not apply in your particular case. In view of individual medical requirements, new research, and government regulations, it is the responsibility of the reader to validate health practices and treatments with a physician or health service.

Acknowledgements

I want to give a huge thanks to my amazing editors Kendra Chun and Sandra K. Friend for their incredibly helpful assistance with putting this book together. I also greatly appreciate my fantastic Creative Director, Rebecca Richards, as well as Letitia Truslow, my wonderful Director of Media Relations. I enjoyed working with all of them and found their help indispensable in creating this exceptional book for women.

Table of Contents

Introduction 6
    The Decline in Estrogen Levels Affects Our Health 8
    My Patient's Concerns about Estrogen Replacement Therapy 10
    Studies Reinforce Women's Concerns About the Safety of HRT 12
    The Purpose of This Book 13
    How to Use This Book 14

Part I: Estrogen - the Incredible Women's Hormone 16

Chapter 1: What is Estrogen? 17
    The Types of Estrogen 17
    How Estrogen Affects the Body 18
    How Estrogen Production Changes Over Our Lifetime 19
    How Diet, Health, and Environmental Estrogens Affect Estrogen Levels 20

Chapter 2: How Estrogen is Produced Within the Body Throughout A Woman's Life 23
    Estrogen Production During Our Active Reproductive Years 23
    Estrogen Production During Premenopause and Perimenopause ... 25
    Estrogen Production After Menopause 26

Chapter 3: Estrogen Deficiency - the Hallmark of Menopause 28
    The Symptoms of Menopause 29
    Is It Menopause? 36
    Testing for Menopause 37

Part II: Healthy Natural Estrogen Therapies 39

Chapter 4: An Introduction to Healthy, Natural Estrogen Therapies 40
    Natural Estrogen Substitutes 41
    Support Your Own Hormones 41
    Understanding Bioidentical Estrogen 42

Chapter 5: Benefit From Estrogen-Like Hormone Substitutes 44
    Estrogen Support with Phyto Foods 44
    The Healing Power of Plants 55
    Restoring the Yin 59
    Vitamins that Reduce Menopause Symptoms 62

Chapter 6: Support Your Own Estrogen Production 65

- Serotonin 66
- Melatonin 69
- Glandulars 71
- Nutrients that Increase Estrogen Production 76
- Nutrients that Decrease the Breakdown and Elimination of Estrogen 77

Chapter 7: Estriol - Your Body's Natural Estrogen 81

- Using Biochemically Identical Estrogen 83

Chapter 8: Estrogen Breakdown and Elimination from the Body 84

- Vitamin B Complex 85
- DIM 85
- D-Glucarate 88
- Limonene 89
- Fiber 90
- Probiotics 91

Part III: How Healthy Lifestyle Supports Estrogen Levels 92

Chapter 9: How Diet Affects Your Estrogen Levels 93

- Foods That Ease Menopausal Symptoms 94
- Foods to Avoid or Limit with Menopause 103

Chapter 10: Managing Stress for Healthy Estrogen Levels 112

- What is Stress? 112
- Stress and Our Bodies 113
- Stress and Estrogen Deficiency 115
- Practice Deep Breathing and Meditation 115
- General Relaxation Exercises 117

Chapter 11: Exercise Supports Healthy Estrogen 122

- Researchers Support Exercise's Medicinal Benefits 122
- Building a Personal Exercise Program to Evaluate Your Fitness Level 125
- Choosing an Exercise Program 125
- Motivating Yourself to Exercise 127
- Beginning an Exercise Program for Menopause 128
- Activities for Menopausal Women 129
- Benefits of Exercise 129

About Susan M. Lark, M.D. 130
Dr. Susan's Solutions Health Library For Women 131
About Womens Wellness Publishing 133

Introduction

Dear Friend,

I know that you are reading this book because you are looking for positive and effective solutions for estrogen therapy. I have written this book just for you, to share with you the all natural treatment program that I have developed and successfully treated thousands of my patients.

As a medical doctor working with many thousands of women patients, I've come to appreciate the wonderful health benefits of estrogen when it is present in proper balance within the body. This powerful hormone, along with our other sex hormones, helps to regulate not only our body chemistry but also physical characteristics such as our skin texture, muscle tone and body shape.

Many tissues and organs in our body are sensitive to and have receptors that bind to estrogen. As a result, estrogen enters the cells of many different tissues and stimulates chemical reactions and physiological changes. Estrogen affects the physical characteristics that we tend to think of as specifically female.

First of all, estrogen causes the growth of our sexual organs. During childhood, we produce estrogen in only small amounts. During puberty, estrogen production increases twentyfold or more. With the increased estrogenic stimulation, female sexual organs begin to change into those of adult women. Our uterus, vagina and fallopian tubes increase in size; our external genitals enlarge. Our vaginal and urinary tract linings thicken and become much more resistant to trauma and infection.

This is important in adulthood when women become sexually active. With estrogen stimulation, the lining of the uterus thickens and the endometrial glands develop—necessary to nourish a fertilized egg during the early stages of pregnancy.

Estrogen has a dramatic effect on the beauty of our skin and hair. Estrogen is responsible for the disposition of fat under the skin, giving rise to the soft and fine-textured skin that many women enjoy during their younger years. It also causes fluid and salt retention in the tissues, which additionally helps to plump up and fill out our skin. When estrogen levels are healthy, our hair tends to be fuller, thicker and shinier.

Finally, estrogen has an important effect on promoting bone health. It helps retain calcium in the bones thereby protecting against bone loss. By reducing the levels of low-density lipoprotein (LDL) in the body and elevating the levels of the protective blood fats, estrogen protects women from developing heart attacks and strokes. These "good" fats are called the high-density lipoproteins (HDL).

In addition, estrogen has a direct positive effect on the endothelial lining of the blood vessels, as well as affecting dozens of other physiological functions as varied as blood sugar level, emotional balance and memory. Clearly, estrogen is crucial to our lives as women and to help us maintain a high level of health and vitality.

The Decline in Estrogen Levels Affects Our Health

As with many positive things in life, we often take them for granted and don't miss them until we lose them. I believe that this is certainly the case with our own production of estrogen. This hormone works silently for several decades, creating incredible support for our body's health and well-being.

Yet, once we reach our forties and fifties (and even thirties for some women) our production of this essential hormone begins to become erratic and finally decrease as much as 75 to 90 percent. This is due to the aging of the ovaries and adrenals, which produce estrogen within the body, as well as the brain and nervous system which help to regulate this process.

What I have seen with my own patients is that when many women enter their menopausal years, it's as if they cross over an invisible line in their lives. As a result of the decline in their estrogen levels, many women often find that their bodies, and therefore, their lives are significantly changed.

While women often complain about menopausal symptoms that are strictly physical, such as vaginal dryness, bladder and vaginal infections, and dryness of the skin—they complain just as often about symptoms that affect their memory, their mood, their job performance, social relationships, and even their ability to take pleasure in day-to-day activities.

I have been amazed by the number of my female patients who begin to complain of forgetfulness and memory loss with the onset of menopause. Small details of life, such as remembering someone's name or where they put the car keys, suddenly become an issue. Competent performance at work is a real concern for some of these women. They report going from one office to another with no idea of why they went there. They may even complain about an inability to recall important work data.

Virtually all of my patients who suffer from forgetfulness and memory loss are concerned about this problem. Some of them wonder if they are in the early stages of senility or even Alzheimer's disease. Fortunately, this is rarely the case. However, the brain is loaded with hormone receptors, and your normal mental and emotional functions depend, in part, on the abundant production of female sex hormones.

While memory loss can affect a woman's competence at work, frequent hot flashes can be downright embarrassing. Women with more severe symptoms may have as many as 10, 20, or even 40 episodes a day. Hot flashes cause a woman to turn pink and either simply generate a lot of heat within the body or perspire profusely. In any case, women often feel like shedding clothes, which is often not possible in a professional setting.

Hot flashes are triggered by stress and often occur at the worst possible times. Some of my patients report having hot flashes while presenting a report in front of a professional audience, in meetings with important customers, or when going for a job interview. Hot flashes also frequently occur at night, waking the woman, and sometimes even her bedmate, from a deep sleep. Frequently interrupted sleep can cause anyone to be tired, irritable, and relatively unproductive the next day.

In addition, the ability to experience joy in life can be blunted by the onset of menopause. Estrogen and other hormones produced by the ovaries and adrenal glands are crucial for maintaining sexual pleasure, a sense of emotional well-being, optimism, and other qualities that women regard as essential for an exciting and satisfying life.

The negative effects of the natural decline in female sex hormone production during menopause are not uncommon. Menopausal symptoms are so common in the United States that 80 to 85 percent of American women experience them to some degree. A small number of these women are lucky enough to have mild symptoms, such as occasional hot flashes over a period of a few months to a year. However, the majority of women have symptoms that are bothersome enough to cause them to seek the help of physicians or to seek solutions on their own by reading books and articles.

My Patient's Concerns about Estrogen Replacement Therapy

Most women who are in menopause are offered conventional estrogen replacement therapy (and often, synthetic progesterone therapy called "progestins") by their physicians or health care provider. For decades, this type of therapy was considered the "gold standard" of care for women suffering from menopause symptoms due to estrogen deficiency.

Yet, in the past ten to fifteen years, landmark research studies have conclusively started to prove the dangers of conventional estrogen replacement therapy (ERT) as well as combination therapy in which synthetic or animal forms of estrogen are combined with synthetic progesterone or progestins hormone replacement therapy (HRT).

The many studies that have followed in the past decade have continued to build the case against these types of therapies. I have been following this research intensively and have had strong concerns regarding physicians' continued persistence in using HRT. Women are also becoming more and more aware of this negative research and, as a result, are becoming more concerned about using these therapies to support their low levels of estrogen. I want to share one of my patient's experiences with you.

> ### Anne's Story
>
> When Anne came to me for a menopause consultation, she placed a newspaper article on my desk about hormone replacement therapy (HRT) and the risk of breast cancer. She was 54 and had fairly severe menopause symptoms, including five to six episodes of hot flashes a day, night sweats two to three times per week, insomnia, anxiety and jitters, and difficulty concentrating. Clearly, she needed help.
>
> Her regular physician recommended that she begin a course of conventional HRT, but she was not enthusiastic about this treatment option. She found it quite upsetting to read about the increased risk of breast cancer with the use of HRT. Her own mother had died of breast cancer at age 60, and she herself had a long history of benign breast disease.
>
> I recommended that she try black cohosh. I have found that for women, like Anne, there are many alternative therapies that can be used to safely and effectively instead of conventional estrogen replacement therapy. These alternative therapies not only provide relief from menopause symptoms, but they do not increase the risk of breast cancer or other health conditions that are an issue with conventional hormone therapy. It was no surprise that Ruth quickly found relief, and, most importantly, peace of mind with this option.

Unlike Anne, who never opted to begin using HRT, many of my patients have come to me, already using conventional hormone therapy. These women have strongly voiced to me their desire to quit using HRT altogether and to begin using safe alternative therapies instead. All of these patients have been concerned about the negative side effects of conventional estrogen therapy or its long-term health consequences.

Their concerns have included fear that ERT would intensify serious preexisting health problems such as bloating, weight gain, breast tenderness, anxiety or depression, heavy bleeding from uterine fibroid tumors, severe migraine headaches, or blood clotting problems.

Other women, free of illness, fear that the long-term use of estrogen may accelerate the onset of a disease for which they are at risk, based on a strong family history, like breast cancer or heart disease. Some of my patients have refused to use estrogen on a philosophical basis, preferring instead to pursue nondrug treatment options such as nutritional therapies and acupuncture.

Studies Reinforce Women's Concerns About the Safety of HRT

My patients have mirrored the fear and concerns of millions of women in the United States. An article that was published in *Family Practice News*, a journal for physicians who are more likely to prescribe conventional estrogen therapy for their patients, stated that there has never been a time in the U.S. when more than 35 percent of menopausal women have opted to use HRT. This reinforces the issue that most physicians prescribe HRT yet relatively few women opt to use it.

Recent studies support these findings with hormone replacement therapy use as low as 8 percent in some parts of the country. The most common reasons women gave for stopping hormone therapy are menstrual-like bleeding, the fear that the increased hormones will increase their risk of developing breast cancer, weight gain and bloating, or ineffectiveness of the therapy to adequately control their symptoms.

Another study of more than 2000 women found that the majority had either ceased using hormones replacement therapy entirely or had significantly cut their originally prescribed dosage. With 80 to 85 percent of all menopausal women symptomatic to some degree, most women could benefit from some type of treatment. However, many women simply don't know about other treatment options available to them, or they are uncertain about the right path to choose to support their estrogen levels.

Unfortunately, women are rarely given alternative therapy options to support their bodies' need for estrogen by their physicians. Conventional physicians commonly prescribed animal-based and synthetic HRT to women as their only option to help stave off hot flashes, night sweats, irritability, and other menopausal symptoms. Few women learn about alternative therapies and even fewer hear how to use lifestyle modification to reduce menopausal symptoms and risk factors for disease from their own health provider. As a result, many women do not get the treatment best suited to their own body's needs.

The Purpose of This Book

I have written this book to help you and other women find the best healthy, natural estrogen treatment options so that your menopause years are symptom free and, even more importantly, so that you remain healthy, strong and vital. My goal is to help you find the safe, natural support your body needs so that you can enjoy life to the fullest.

To help you develop the best estrogen support program for yourself, I included in this book much of the information that I have shared with women who have seen me as patients or attended my classes. I have been delighted to see so many of my patients become symptom free and benefit greatly from the programs that I have created for them.

I discuss the estrogen supportive benefits of a wide variety of foods, vitamins, minerals, herbs, essential fatty acids, and bioidentical estrogen replacement therapy, as well as, how to detoxify and eliminate estrogen from the body so that your estrogen levels remain in healthy balance. I also share with you helpful information on how stress reduction and aerobic exercise can support healthy estrogen levels.

Each woman dealing with estrogen deficiency issues due to menopause has her own unique set of symptoms and her own concerns. I have found working with my own patients that there is no "one size fits all" solution to this issue. Each woman needs a customized program that suits her own needs. That is why I have shared with you a wide variety of options for you to choose from.

While reading this book, I recommend that you try the natural estrogen options that most appeal to you and are consistent with your current lifestyle, beliefs and philosophy of care. Above all, remember that information contained in this book is presented to help you make educated choices about your health care needs. When you are knowledgeable and informed, you are far more likely to make choices that will bring you symptom relief and better health. The midlife years and beyond can be exciting and fulfilling when you participate actively in your health care decisions.

After reading this book, be sure to share with your health care practitioner any questions you have about estrogen replacement therapy or other therapies. If you do not feel that your doctor is receptive to your concerns and questions, you may want to find another practitioner in your community with whom you feel more comfortable.

Ideally, doctor and patient should work together as a team on the patient's behalf, implementing the best solutions for the patient's health care problems. To achieve this goal, you may have to assume an active role and take responsibility for letting your physician know that you wish to participate in the process of making decisions about your health and well-being. You may also need to convey that it is important to you to have meaningful dialogue about your health issues.

How to Use This Book

This book is divided into three parts to make it easy and effective to use. Part I contains chapters on important facts about estrogen as well as how we produce and metabolize estrogen in our bodies and how this process changes as we go through menopause. I discuss the symptoms of menopause that occur as the levels of estrogen begin to diminish at midlife; provide you with a very helpful menopause questionnaire to chart your symptoms; and, finally, I discuss testing for estrogen levels in the body to determine your hormonal status.

In Part II, I share vital information about healthy, natural estrogen therapies including foods, vitamins, minerals, herbs, essential fatty acids and bioidentical estrogen therapy that can be used as a safe and effective alternative to conventional ERT. These safe, natural alternative therapies either provide you with estrogen-like support, help to create healthier estrogen levels within your own body after menopause or act as bioidentical estrogen replacement therapy.

In Part III, I discuss the best dietary choices to maintain healthier estrogen levels, and, to support your health in general after menopause. I also discuss the estrogen support benefits of stress reduction and regular aerobic exercise.

I hope that you enjoy working with the information and therapies on healthy, natural estrogen contained in this book and that your midlife and older years are symptom free, healthy and full of energy and vitality!

Love,

Dr. Susan

Part I:
Estrogen - the Incredible Women's Hormone

1

What is Estrogen?

In this chapter, I share with you very useful and important information about estrogen. This information will help you understand the crucial role that estrogen plays in our bodies and why it is so important to maintain our level of estrogen after menopause.

You will learn about the different types of estrogen that we produce in our bodies; how estrogen affects the body; how estrogen production changes over our lifetime; the health benefits of estrogen; and, finally, how diet, health, and the environment affect estrogen levels.

The Types of Estrogen

Estrogen, along with progesterone, is one of the two major hormones that support the functioning of the female reproductive organs and the menstrual cycle. The ovaries and adrenal glands produce substantial amounts of estrogen during a woman's active reproductive years and continue to produce small amounts after menopause. While we are accustomed to using the term estrogen, this term actually refers to several different types of estrogens made within the body.

At least six types of estrogen have been identified and are classified according to their potency. The term potency refers to the time that estrogen is bound to the estrogen receptor within a specific tissue. The higher the estrogen potency, the more time it remains bound to the receptor site. As a result, the physiological effects that estrogen promotes within that tissue are more pronounced. For example, estrogen is a growth-stimulating hormone, causing tissues to grow and thicken; it also causes water and salt to be retained within the tissues of the body. The more potent and powerful forms of estrogen cause these effects to occur in a more pronounced fashion.

The three main types of estrogen produced within the body are estradiol, estrone, and estriol. Estradiol is the most potent form of estrogen. It is the primary type of estrogen produced by the ovaries during a woman's reproductive years. Estrone is an intermediate-potency form of estrogen, 12 times weaker than estradiol. It is mainly produced within the fatty tissue of the body from precursor hormones made by the adrenal glands. Obviously, the more weight a woman carries, the more adrenal estrogen she is capable of making. Small amounts of estrone are also produced by the ovaries after menopause, when production of estradiol ceases.

As estradiol and estrone circulate through the body, they pass through the liver. It is the liver's job to detoxify and metabolize these two estrogens to a weaker form, which can then be eliminated from the body. Since estrogen is constantly being produced by the ovaries and adrenal glands, the liver helps to prevent its accumulation to toxic levels. Estriol, the liver metabolite of the other two estrogens, is the weakest form of estrogen produced by the body. It is 80 times weaker than estradiol.

How Estrogen Affects the Body

The effect that estrogen has on a woman's body begins even before birth, since estrogen plays an important role in the development of female sexual characteristics. During childhood, a girl's body produces only small amounts of estrogen. Then, at puberty, when estrogen production increases twenty-fold or more, these higher levels stimulate the female sexual organs of young girls to begin to mature into those of an adult woman.

Estrogen causes the uterus and vagina to increase in size. It stimulates the vagina and urinary tract linings to thicken and become more resistant to trauma and infection, thus preparing a woman to eventually become sexually active and bear children. In addition, estrogen causes an increase in overall body fat, contributing to the softly rounded female contours that we associate with sexual maturation. Firm, youthful-looking skin is also attributable to estrogen, which stimulates collagen, a protein that makes up 90 percent of the skin. Estrogen promotes the growth of pubic hair and coloration of the nipples and also stimulates bone growth. Beginning at puberty, when estrogen production soars, a young woman's height also rapidly increases.

The various actions of estrogen are balanced by the complementary effects of progesterone. These two hormones, working together, help regulate a notably wide range of physiological processes. For instance, estrogen decreases the level of oxygen in cells, and progesterone restores oxygen to normal levels. While estrogen increases body fat, progesterone helps the body burn fat for energy. Estrogen also promotes salt and fluid retention, whereas progesterone is a natural diuretic, increasing the flow of urine. Estrogen promotes blood clotting, while progesterone normalizes clotting. Furthermore, estrogen impairs blood sugar control, and progesterone normalizes blood sugar levels. When these hormones are in balance, they provide a host of health benefits.

How Estrogen Production Changes Over Our Lifetime

The amount of estrogen a woman produces changes during her lifetime. The normal output of estradiol is 100 to 300 mg. a day.

Estrogen is also produced in pregnancy by the placenta (a spongy structure in the uterus, from which the fetus derives oxygen and nourishment). The placenta produces estrogen in great quantity, as much as 100 times the amount normally made by the ovaries.

Levels of estrogen tend to fluctuate during the month because of menstruation, with it reaching peak levels during the first half of the menstrual cycle. During the second half of the cycle, both estrogen and progesterone are produced, though estrogen production does decline somewhat from its levels earlier in the month.

With the onset of menopause, after menstruation has ceased entirely, ovarian production of estrogen is greatly reduced, and levels of circulating estrogen decline by as much as 75 to 90 percent. However, after menopause, one-fourth to one-third of all American women continue to make enough ovarian and adrenal estrogen in its weaker form, estrone. While the quantity produced is not enough to cause a monthly menstrual cycle, it is sufficient to support the health of tissues such as bone, skin, and the vaginal lining.

Although being overweight is a liability for many health conditions, those women who have more fatty tissue are better able to convert androgens (male hormones) to estrone after menopause. Consequently, they tend to have stronger bones and more youthful-looking skin. The women who maintain estrogen production after menopause probably do not need to consider hormone replacement therapy for ten to fifteen more years. The majority of women, however, have an abrupt decline in their estrogen production to the point that uncomfortable symptoms will lead these women to seek medical care.

Benefits of Estrogen

- Prevents menopausal symptoms
- Increases physical vitality and stamina
- Protects against heart disease and stroke
- Prevents osteoporosis and joint disease
- Enhances mental clarity and acuity

How Diet, Health, and Environmental Estrogens Affect Estrogen Levels

While estrogen production declines with age, the amount of estrogen in the body will also be influenced by a range of other factors, including diet, digestive capabilities, liver function, enzyme levels, and exposure to environmental toxins--a topic that has not received sufficient attention to date.

Diet

Meat, poultry, and dairy foods contain estrogens that have been injected into the animals to fatten them for market. One of the synthetic estrogens routinely given to livestock was DES (diethylstilbestrol). DES was also given to women to prevent miscarriages and symptoms of menopause, until it was associated with birth defects in their offspring and was finally banned in 1979. However, today poultry and livestock, especially dairy cows, are still given other forms of estrogen compounds. Hormones such as estrogen accumulate in fatty tissue in the animals we eat as well as in us, and high-fat diets have been associated with changes in human estrogen levels.

Caffeine and alcohol consumption can also influence estrogen levels. Excessive alcohol intake can affect the liver's ability to break down estrogen for excretion. This elevates the body's blood estrogen levels, particularly of the more chemically active forms of estrogen that have been linked to diseases like breast cancer. A three-year study appearing in the *American Journal of Epidemiology*, involving 728 white, postmenopausal females aged 42 to 90, found that caffeine intake had an effect on estrogen levels. Having more than two cups of coffee or four cans of caffeinated soda per day increased blood levels of this hormone.

Another research study suggested that a diet high in sugar may impair liver function, affecting its ability to metabolize estrogen. Even the public water supply may contain estrogens. Water that is recycled at treatment plants may still contains traces of excreted synthetic estrogens such as those contained in birth control pills that would have been excreted from the bodies of women using these products.

Physiological Factors

Poor digestive function can prevent hormone precursors such as fat molecules from being absorbed. Problems with the liver can also lead to low levels of hormones. Persons with functional disorders of the liver have been shown to have low levels of estrogen. When liver enzyme systems are impaired and the detoxification function is inadequate, the quantity and quality of hormone formation is reduced. Depressed levels of HDL cholesterol can also lead to lower levels of estrogen, as this deficiency blocks the biochemical pathway required for the production of the primary precursor hormone, pregnenolone, and all the consequent sex hormones, including estrogen, progesterone, and testosterone.

Environmental Estrogens

Pollutants that have estrogen-like activity when they are taken into the body (xenoestrogens) can wreak havoc on our own estrogen function.

These substances are found in an enormous range of products for the home and workplace. They are present in cosmetics, detergents and dishwashing liquids, and bug spray. Pesticides and industrial chemicals such as organochlorines, dioxins, and PCBs (polychlorinated biphenyls) also contain substances related to estrogen.

A study from Stanford University, published in the *Journal of the American Medical Association*, noted that when polycarbonate plastics are heated, they release bisphenol-A, a substance that is known to have estrogenic activity. Microwaving foods in plastic containers or using a plastic cup for hot coffee can cause estrogen substances to leech into the food.

There are many suspected health consequences of our wide exposure to xenoestrogens, including an increased risk of PMS and breast cancer. This problem has also affected male reproductive health, and has been implycated in lowering sperm counts in men all over the world.

According to a study published in the *British Medical Journal*, there has been a clear decline in the average sperm count worldwide during the last 50 years. The researchers conducted an analysis of 61 papers that involved a total of 14,947 men. When the results were compared, the researchers found that the average sperm count had decreased by nearly half from the late 1930's to the early 1990's. A further study, published in *The Lancet*, found that the multiplication of sertoli cells, which are responsible for sperm production, is inhibited by estrogen.

2

How Estrogen is Produced Within the Body Throughout A Woman's Life

In this chapter, I discuss with you the science behind the intricate feedback system that creates estrogen within our bodies. When this system is working well, our estrogen levels are healthy and support our bodies well. However, when this system begins to work less efficiently, as we enter our mid to late thirties, forties, fifties and beyond, our health profile begins to shift, also. If you would like to skip this material about the science of estrogen production, you may go on to the next chapter.

Estrogen Production During Our Active Reproductive Years

During our younger years, when we are having regular menstrual periods, estrogen is produced each month through a feedback system that operates between our ovaries, which actually produces estrogen, and the hormones manufactured by the brain that regulate this system.

This intricate feedback system causes our levels of estrogen to fluctuate throughout the month. When the ovaries secrete high levels of estrogen and progesterone, this "turns off" production of hypothalamic and pituitary hormones, which are produced within the brain, that normally stimulate ovarian function. Conversely, when ovarian production of estrogen and progesterone are low, the hypothalamic and pituitary hormone production rises in an attempt to stimulate the ovaries to work harder.

How does the feedback system operate in the menstrual cycle? The initial trigger for the menstrual cycle comes from hormones produced in the hypothalamus, a walnut-sized collection of highly specialized brain cells located above the pituitary. The hypothalamus regulates many basic bodily functions in addition to the production of female sex hormones, including temperature control, sleep patterns, thirst and hunger. The hypothalamus is very sensitive to stress such as emotional problems and infections. Severe stress can affect the ability of the hypothalamus to pass signals to the pituitary and on to the other endocrine glands. This can cause an imbalance in the menstrual cycle.

The pituitary, located at the base of the brain, stimulates all the glands of the body and provides the next mechanism that regulates the menstrual cycle. To communicate with the pituitary, the hypothalamus releases messengers into the bloodstream called FSH-RF (follicle-stimulating hormone-releasing factor) and LH-RF (luteinizing hormone-releasing factor). When these messages from the hypothalamus are received, the pituitary begins to produce its own hormones which trigger the menstrual cycle and ovulation by secreting FSH (follicle-stimulating hormone) and LH (luteinizing hormone).

Once FSH and LH are released into the bloodstream, their destinations are the ovaries, the female reproductive organ. The ovaries are two small, almond-shaped glands located in a woman's pelvis. The ovaries hold all the eggs a woman will ever have, in an inactive form called follicles. At birth, each female may have as many as 1 million follicles. By puberty, the number of eggs has been reduced to 300,000 to 400,000. The eggs decrease in number throughout a woman's life, until menopause, at which time the follicles have atrophied and lost their ability to produce estrogen. Without sufficient estrogen, menstruation ceases.

Each month, FSH and LH from the pituitary cause the follicles to ripen and the release of an egg for possible fertilization. (Usually, only one ovary is stimulated in a cycle.) As this occurs, the follicles begin to produce the hormones estrogen and progesterone. Estrogen reaches its peak during the first half of the cycle, while progesterone output occurs after midcycle when ovulation has occurred.

After midcycle, usually around day 14 in a 28-day cycle, ovulation occurs. Ovulation refers to the production of a mature egg cell which is capable of being fertilized. Normally, the mature egg finds its way to a fallopian tube for the journey to the uterus. The follicle that produced the egg for that month (or Graafian follicle) is further stimulated after midcycle by LH and changes into the yellow body, or corpus luteum. The corpus luteum secretes progesterone, the second ovarian hormone of the menstrual cycle. Progesterone helps prepare the uterine lining for a possible pregnancy.

If the egg is fertilized, it will implant on the uterine wall and the corpus luteum will continue to secrete progesterone. If no fertilization occurs, the corpus luteum begins to deteriorate and the progesterone and estrogen levels decrease. The lining of the uterus starts to break down and menstruation begins. With the onset of menstruation, the monthly ebb and flow of hormones begins again.

Estrogen Production During Premenopause and Perimenopause

As women reach their early forties, the reproductive tract begins to show signs of aging. By this time, most women have ovulated regularly for almost 30 years. With each ovulation, one follicle matures for a possible pregnancy. However, an additional 1000 follicles or more degenerate with each menstrual cycle and lose their ability to be fertilized. At this rate, most women have exhausted their supply of follicles by their late forties or early fifties.

As the number of follicles diminishes, the remaining follicles produce less estrogen. During the cycles when the follicles don't mature to ovulation, progesterone production is insufficient or absent. In fact, during the transition to menopause, ovulation occurs with decreasing frequency. Because of this drop in hormonal output by the ovaries, the pituitary hormone FSH rises in an attempt to drive the ovary to secrete more estrogen. Sometimes the high levels of FSH can over stimulate the remaining follicles to produce an abundance of estrogen. In such cycles, a woman may produce very high levels of estrogen yet not produce progesterone because the follicles never mature sufficiently. The tendency for estrogen to fluctuate between low and high levels of production can continue throughout the menopause transition and may last from one to seven years.

During this time, women are very vulnerable to developing a variety of health problems. The imbalance in the estrogen and progesterone levels can trigger the growth of uterine fibroids, PMS symptoms and changes in the amount and frequency of the menstrual cycle. Women whose estrogen level drops tend to have longer intervals between periods, with lighter bleeding, before stopping entirely. Women who have temporary surges in estrogen levels prior to menopause without the secretion of progesterone may have increasingly heavy and more frequent menstrual bleeding. The menstrual cycle often becomes irregular.

This can be a very difficult time for some women and they are faced with the need for close monitoring by their physician when symptoms are severe. These symptoms can include heavy menstrual bleeding or the growth of fibroid tumors which may lead to an increased number of hysterectomies in this age group.

Finally, as the follicles become exhausted, the estrogen drops to a level at which there is not enough of this hormone to build up the lining of the uterus sufficiently to induce menstruation. A woman is officially considered to be menopausal when she has had no menstrual period for at least twelve months. For most women, this occurs between the ages of 46 to 53. Some women, however, may experience menopause as early as their thirties or as late as age 59; the average age is 51.

As estrogen levels diminish, the level of FSH begins to rise, finally attaining levels considered to be diagnostic for menopause. FSH continues to remain high during the postmenopausal years. In fact, physicians often monitor FSH levels to determine the onset of menopause.

Estrogen Production After Menopause

During the postmenopausal years, the body does continue to produce small amounts of estrogen. Even though the follicles are exhausted, another part of the ovary called the stroma can still make small amounts of estrogen. The stroma is the supportive tissue of the ovary that helps provide structure to the gland. In addition, the body can also make estrogen by converting the male precursor hormone, androstenedione, to estrogen.

Though androstenedione is made by the adrenal glands, its conversion to estrogen occurs in the body's fat cells. Obese women make more estrogen after menopause because they have more fat cells. In fact, some women may make enough estrogen to delay aging of the skin, vagina, bladder, breasts, and other tissue for a decade or so. Thinner women tend to show loss of estrogen support earlier, as do women with less active adrenal or ovarian stromal output of hormones.

By the time women reach their seventies and eighties, however, even these small extra sources of estrogen begin to diminish. As the hormonal support falls to lower and lower levels, the female body gradually ages during the years following menopause.

In the early postmenopausal years, common symptoms of diminished hormonal output include hot flashes, night sweats, vaginal and bladder atrophy, mood swings and fatigue. The lack of hormonal support can increase the risk of osteoporosis, heart attacks, adverse lipid and vessel wall changes, and stroke. These symptoms and health issues will be discussed in depth in the following chapter.

Not all women produce the same amounts and/or types of estrogen after menopause. Because androstenedione is converted into estrone in your fatty tissues, women with more body fat have more circulating estrogen than thin women. Additionally, in my clinical practice, have found that women with better nutrition habits and women who are less stressed and more relaxed have healthier estrogen balance and make more estrogen than women who don't watch their food intake and stress levels. If you are one of these lucky women—and you can be with my program—then you will experience significantly fewer menopausal symptoms, have more energy, and sail through the transition in comfort.

3

Estrogen Deficiency - the Hallmark of Menopause

Somewhere between the ages of 43 and 59 years old, most women will usually begin to experience fewer and fewer monthly menstrual periods, and bleeding becomes scanter and scanter. You may also experience hot flashes and other menopause-like symptoms. This is considered the perimenopause phase. Eventually, you will cease menstruation altogether, with the cessation of a menstrual period for 12 straight months signaling the official start of menopause.

Once your periods have stopped completely, you are considered postmenopausal. At this point, estrogen production will have dropped 75 to 90 percent. This life change is due to normal aging of ovaries and egg follicles. Your ovaries and adrenal glands continue to produce a small amount of estradiol (the most potent form of estrogen) and estrone (a middle potency estrogen), and the liver produces some estriol (the weakest form of estrogen). While the action of estrone and estriol is not nearly as strong as the estrogen produced before menopause, these hormones do continue to provide some support for the bones, heart, vagina, and other tissues.

There are two different types of menopause. The first type is experienced by most women. It is natural and typically occurs between the ages of 43 and 59. Though the average age for the onset of menopause is 51 years, some women can begin the change in their mid- to late-40's (early-onset) or not until their early-60's (late-onset). About 12.5 percent of women experience early-onset menopause, and this pattern often runs in a woman's family. Menopause is considered to be late-onset if it occurs after age 55. In fact, less than one percent of women continue menstruating after age 59.

The second type of menopause is "artificial", meaning that something outside of a woman's natural physiology triggered menopause. Many women who experience menopause in their 30's and 40's fall into this category.

The two most common causes of artificial menopause are chemotherapy and hysterectomy. The chemicals used in cancer chemotherapy can, and often do, interfere with your ovaries' ability to produce estrogen. I have had a number of women in my clinical practice that ceased menstruation in their early to late thirties and forties because of chemotherapy for breast cancer.

In the case of hysterectomy, you will always have cessation of periods, but you may or may not still produce your normal levels of hormones. This depends on whether or not you still have your ovaries. If you had only your uterus removed but still have your ovaries, then the surgery will probably not trigger the actual symptoms of hormone deficiency commonly seen with menopause, although hormone levels often fluctuate or even diminish due to the stress of the surgery.

If you've had a hysterectomy that involved the removal of your ovaries as well as your uterus, then your ability to produce hormones has been greatly compromised. Since your ovaries have been removed, your entire hormone production has been drastically reduced, and all of your hormone production is now dependent upon your adrenals. Plus, the shock of the surgery itself may further reduce your adrenals' ability to produce hormones. As a result, menopause symptoms such as hot flashes and vaginal dryness are often experienced almost immediately following this type of surgery.

The Symptoms of Menopause

For many women in menopause, this time of life brings a number of uncomfortable symptoms, usually due to the diminished production of estrogen. In addition to the commonly known hot flashes and night sweats, menopause can bring a whole host of physical, mental, and emotional changes primarily due to a deficiency of estrogen, as well as the other sex hormones.

Hot Flashes / Night Sweats

As many as 85 percent of all menopausal women in the United States experience some degree of hot flashes. Women with more severe symptoms may have as many as 10, 20, or even 40 episodes a day, while other women may only experience them a few times a week or during times of stress. The episodes are the result of increased blood flow to the brain, organs, and skin, causing a sudden sensation of warmth that may be followed by chills. On average, a hot flash lasts about two to five minutes. Most experts agree that hot flashes are caused by either an abrupt withdrawal of estrogen or a sudden increase in the neurotransmitter norepinephrine.

Hot flashes are physically draining, since your body loses fluids and minerals in the process of perspiring. And if they occur at the workplace or during social functions, they can be embarrassing. When they take the form of night sweats, hot flashes may disrupt sleep and soak sheets, leaving you cranky and exhausted. Hot flashes cause a woman to turn pink and either perspire profusely or simply generate a lot of heat within the body. In any case, women often feel like shedding clothes, which is usually not possible in a professional setting.

Fortunately, hot flashes don't last forever. About 50 percent of women see relief within a year. For another 30 percent, hot flashes can last two or three years. And for an uncomfortable 20 percent of women, hot flashes can linger for 5 to 10 years.

Insomnia

A number of studies have shown that estrogen decreases the frequency of awakenings during the night and increases the amount of restorative rapid eye movement (REM) sleep, the type of sleep that occurs when a person is dreaming, which is necessary for feeling rested the next day.

When estrogen levels are deficient, you are likely to sleep more fitfully and for fewer hours. Lacking adequate sleep, you are more likely to feel tired during the day. If you have had an abrupt decline in your estrogen levels by undergoing gynecological surgery, including the removal of your uterus and/or ovaries, you may suffer more acutely from interrupted sleep.

Loss of Libido

When estrogen decreases, vaginal tissues begin to atrophy and your natural lubricants decrease. Your vagina then becomes gradually thinner and less elastic. This can cause intercourse to be painful, and you may experience soreness after sex. Pain during intercourse can also increase your reluctance to have sex.

After menopause, your production of testosterone and other androgens (male hormones) also decline. These hormones normally stimulate sex drive. While androgens are produced throughout your cycle, during your active reproductive years, their levels increase before mid-cycle, thereby increasing your desire for sex just as an egg is ready to be fertilized.

When everything is working perfectly, you have a healthy desire for sex. But as your body shifts gears during the transition to menopause, desire tends to decrease. And while some testosterone still cycles in your bloodstream, the amount may be insufficient to spark desire.

Osteoporosis

Throughout most of your life, your female hormones work to build bone, even as calcium and other alkaline minerals are drawn out of your bones to prevent over-acidity and support the healthy, slightly alkaline pH of your blood.

After menopause, your body continues to draw on your bones' alkaline mineral reserves, but bone building is greatly diminished, due to the significant decline of your female hormone production. The result is more porous, fragile, and brittle bones. Older women with osteoporosis have lost as much as 40 to 45 percent of their total bone mass. In fact, statistics from the National Osteoporosis Foundation indicate that osteoporosis is responsible for 1.5 million fractures each year, and affects more than 20 million women. Fortunately, bone can be rebuilt with my estrogen support program, the right diet, supplements, and exercise.

Heart Disease and Stroke

The incidence of heart disease escalates as women age and estrogen production declines. Estrogen is known to help keep the arteries clear of plaque. From age 30 to 60, cancer is the main cause of death in women, with heart disease ranking second for women age 40 to 60. However, after age 60, heart disease becomes the leading cause of death in American women, claiming the lives of nearly 500,000 women each year, and affecting another three million.

Current research shows that the relationship between estrogen and heart disease is tied to estrogen's role in maintaining healthy cholesterol levels, namely keeping the "good" high-density lipoprotein (HDL) levels elevated. Other research indicates that estrogen increases nitric oxide (NO) levels. This gas naturally inhibits muscle contraction and helps to relax blood vessels. As a result, it helps to promote blood flow and vascular relaxation, and works to make tissues firmer and more elastic.

Vaginal Infections and Dryness

Estrogen causes the uterus and vagina to increase in size. It stimulates the vagina and urinary tract linings to thicken and become more resistant to trauma and infection, thus preparing a woman to eventually become sexually active and bear children. When estrogen decreases, vaginal tissues begin to atrophy and your natural lubricants decrease. These changes can make you more susceptible to vaginal and bladder infections.

If you experience pain during sex or acquire an infection as a result of intercourse, you may be reluctant to have sex. Your doctor may prescribe drugs for infections, but you must be willing to reveal the full range of your symptoms, including lack of sexual desire, to ensure that you get the best treatment available.

Loss of Skin Tone

Estrogen causes an increase in overall body fat, contributing to the softly rounded female contours that we associate with sexual maturation. Firm, youthful-looking skin is also attributable to estrogen, which stimulates collagen, a protein that makes up 90 percent of the skin. Finally, estrogen causes fluid and sodium retention within the tissue, so your skin is plumper and more hydrated.

To this point, research has found that both the amount of collagen and the thickness of your skin decrease by one to two percent each year following menopause. Fortunately, estrogen substitutes and key herbs and nutrients have been found to prevent collagen atrophy, and even restore decreased thickness.

Mental Confusion

The ability to concentrate and remember details depends, in part, on having adequate amounts of estrogen. As a woman's own estrogen production begins to diminish, cognitive function can decline.

I regularly hear complaints from my menopausal patients of muddled thinking, brain fog, and poor memory. When short-term memory fades, a person may misplace their car keys, forget a friend's name, or even enter a room or office at work with no idea of why they went there.

As estrogen replacement therapy became more popular in the 1960's and 1970's, researchers began to study the effects of hormones on cognitive function in young and middle-aged women. In a review article on estrogen and memory done at McGill University, the researcher found that there is a strong indication that estrogen does help to maintain short- and long-term memory in women. These benefits were noted in verbal recall, but not in visual/spatial memory.

Another study published in *Psychoneuroendocrinology* investigated the effects of estrogen on memory function in women with surgically induced menopause. Nineteen women who were scheduled for hysterectomy and removal of the ovaries were given verbal memory tests before surgery, and again two months after their operation. Postoperatively, the women were treated with either 10 mg of estrogen or a placebo. Memory scores of those women treated with estrogen showed no decline after surgery, whereas the scores of those women who received the placebo declined significantly.

Mood Swings

Your emotions are determined, in part, by your estrogen levels. Because estrogen is a natural stimulant, with a mood-elevating effect, fluctuating estrogen levels can cause emotions to go haywire. When estrogen levels are elevated, a woman may experience anxiety and irritability, while a deficiency of estrogen can lead to depression.

With the decline in estrogen production that occurs during menopause, many women notice that their moods may fluctuate. Some of my patients have complained about mood swings varying between increased anxiety and irritability to depression and fatigue. They have reported being bad tempered toward family, friends, and co-workers and responding to daily-life stresses in a more irritable fashion, similar to the emotional ups and downs of PMS.

Although menopause does not inevitably cause depression, some women do become despondent and gloomy as hormone production declines. Research has shown that supplemental estrogen has a mood-elevating effect. Women on some type of hormone replacement therapy may perceive this effect as an enhanced sense of well-being and overall mental balance, which contributes to the relief of other menopausal symptoms such as hot flashes and vaginal dryness. In a study published in *Clinical Obstetrics and Gynecology*, women were given 1.25 mg daily of either hormone replacement therapy or a placebo for a period of two months. The women were assessed for their degree of irritability and anxiety. Those who received the estrogen treatment reported feeling calmer and more balanced moods with longer periods of well-being.

> **Lorraine's Story**
>
> Several years back, my patient Lorraine was telling me about her experience with menopause. At 53, she had debilitating hot flashes and a loss of sex drive. She had terrible insomnia and searing heartburn. These symptoms affected her career, home life, and relationships.
>
> She tried many different approaches to deal with her symptoms, starting with Premarin—the most frequently prescribed synthetic hormone replacement therapy. It not only made her hot flashes worse, but it also caused nausea and facial swelling. Finally, Lorraine settled on bioidentical estrogen therapy combined with natural progesterone cream. At my suggestion, she also began using the herb kava root for sleep and sodium bicarbonate (baking soda) and peppermint tea for her heartburn. She was eventually able to find relief with this program.

Lorraine's difficulty in finding relief underscores for me the problem many women have at midlife. Finding a menopause solution that works for you must be individualized. The bottom line is you don't have to feel miserable or accept the idea that it's all downhill from here. Menopause may be a hormone-deficiency state, but with the right dietary support, nutritional supplements, and lifestyle changes, you can write your own ticket to good health and well-being after midlife.

Is It Menopause?

The following checklist can help you determine if you are estrogen deficient. If you answered yes to four or more of these questions, you are very likely in menopause.

- My last period was 12 months or longer ago
- My periods are lighter, less frequent, and of shorter duration (late perimenopause)
- I'm 46 or older
- I'm having hot flashes
- Intercourse is painful
- My desire for sex has faded
- I have difficulty achieving orgasm
- I have frequent vaginal infections
- I leak urine when I laugh, cough, sneeze, exercise, or wait too long to void
- I've lost my zest for life
- I have difficulty sleeping through the night
- I'm frequently tired
- I'm anxious and irritable
- I forget small details
- My skin is drier, thinner, and more wrinkled
- My muscles are losing their tone
- I'm gaining weight
- My joints and/or muscles ache
- I have itchy, crawly skin
- I sometimes feel as if electric shocks were going through my body

If you are concerned that this sounds like you, then the next step is to get your hormone levels tested.

Testing for Menopause

The method for checking women's hormone levels had severe limitations until the 1990's. A single blood sample was taken and analyzed, though the results of this one-time check were disgracefully unhelpful. In addition, the stress of having blood drawn was enough to throw off a woman's hormone levels and skew the results.

Fortunately, there are saliva female hormone tests that are non-invasive (no needle sticks!) and highly accurate. These tests can take the guesswork out of making a proper diagnosis and make it possible to design individualized treatment that delivers maximum benefit with minimum risk of side effects.

Best of all, saliva hormone testing is accessible. Even physicians who still don't routinely order saliva hormone testing will usually write an order when a patient requests it. You can even order a limited saliva hormone test kit on your own directly from a laboratory, without a doctor's order.

Saliva Versus Blood

Like blood, saliva closely mirrors hormone levels in your body's tissues. However, saliva is a particularly accurate indicator of free (unbound) hormone levels. This is the key, as only free hormones are active, meaning that they can affect the hormone-sensitive tissues in your breasts, brain, heart, and uterus. Saliva testing therefore provides a superior measure of the levels of hormones that actually affect vital body systems, mood, tissue levels of sodium and fluid, and many other important functions.

Additionally, blood testing only provides a one-time "snapshot" of hormone levels, whereas saliva testing provides a dynamic picture of hormonal ebb and flow over an entire menstrual cycle. In fact, 11 samples are collected during the month, all at the same time of day, then sent to a laboratory. The lab measures and charts your progesterone and estradiol (your most prevalent and potent form of estrogen) levels. These results are then compared to normal patterns.

Finally, saliva testing is easy, stress-free and non-invasive. You can collect your own saliva samples, which means you don't have to go to your doctor's office or a lab. Plus, there's no need to draw blood.

Get Tested

If you think saliva hormone testing is right for you, consider consulting your physician. Having your doctor order the test has two advantages: The profile is more extensive, and your insurance may cover the cost. Several laboratories perform the test; in the event your physician does not have a preference, I recommend Genova Diagnostics (gdx.net or 800-522-4762), as well as ZRT Laboratory (zrtlab.com or 866-600-1636). If your doctor doesn't order the test, or you simply want insight to help you develop your own self-care regimen, you can order a test kit from several sources. Aeron Laboratories has a wonderful Life Cycles saliva test kit (aeron.com or 800-631-7900).

When you get your test results, you'll want to pay particular attention to your estradiol levels. A reading of one to two picograms per milliliter (pg/ml) indicates that you are menopausal.

Have your General Health Checked

I also recommend a full checkup at menopause, including a Pap smear, pelvic and breast exam, and blood tests for liver function, blood sugar, cholesterol, thyroid function, anemia, bone density, and calcium and phosphorous levels. Physicians may also choose to order test levels of the pituitary hormones FSH and LH.

In the following chapters, I discuss the natural, healthy estrogen replacement options available to you. Fortunately, there are many safe and effective treatment options that will not only ease and even prevent menopausal symptoms, but can also protect you from heart disease and breast cancer.

Part II:
Healthy Natural Estrogen Therapies

4

An Introduction to Healthy, Natural Estrogen Therapies

Now that you are aware of the dangerous side effects associated with conventional HRT, you may be wondering what options you do have. Hot flashes, insomnia, lapses in memory and concentration, mood swings, anxiety, night sweats, and the idea of thinning bones are health issues that no woman should have to endure. Fortunately, you don't. There are many safer and very effective nutritional and dietary therapies that have been proven to be very effective, as well as bioidentical estrogen replacement therapy that I will be discussing in this part of the book.

In the years I have been a physician, I've been very impressed by the effectiveness of these safe, natural hormone replacement options. Many thousands of women I've treated have breezed through menopause risk-free and symptom-free by using a combination of natural therapies.

Specifically, there are three main approaches to replacing and enhancing your own natural estrogen. The first involves the use of natural substances such as phytochemicals, herbs, and vitamins that provide estrogenic-like support and even act as estrogen mimics. These are nonprescription, self-care treatment options that can be acquired in health food stores and pharmacies without a doctor's prescription. The second is to support your own "brand" of estrogen and bring you into better hormonal balance within your own body. The third option involves the use of biochemically identical estrogen, which is prescribed by your physician from a compounding pharmacy.

Regardless of which option you select, all of these complementary treatments are gentle, yet highly effective. Let's take a quick look at each category so you can have a better understanding of how each of them works.

Natural Estrogen Substitutes

You can gain an estrogen-like effect from certain foods, nutrients, and herbs. Foods such as soybeans and flaxseed contain phytoestrogens, which are chemically and functionally similar to estradiol, a woman's most prominent natural estrogen.

Nutrients such as bioflavonoids and vitamins A and C have also been shown to mimic estrogen in the body. These compounds are particularly beneficial in relieving hot flashes and vaginal dryness, as well as headaches and irritability.

Finally, herbs like black cohosh and dong quai have been used for centuries to treat abnormal menstruation and alleviate menopausal symptoms. These and other similar herbs—both Western and Chinese—work by stimulating receptors in the pituitary gland and the hypothalamus.

Support Your Own Hormones

Providing support for your own hormone production is a very beneficial approach for women in menopause. I have had wonderful success using my safe, gentle, and effective program to help women accomplish this goal.

My estrogen support program involves the use of specific nutritional supplements and dietary changes, stress reduction, and exercise. In terms of nutrients, I focus on those that either support your own production and levels of hormones or stimulate hormone production. To support production, it's critical to increase your levels of key nutrients that sustain your own estrogen levels. I describe these nutrients in detail later on in this book.

In order to stimulate estrogen, or any sex hormone, production, you also need to boost the health and vitality of those body systems that play key roles in the creation and regulation of the hormones themselves. These include the central nervous system, hypothalamus, ovaries, pituitary and adrenal glands, and your liver, as well as other organs. This can go a long way towards supporting your hormones safely, naturally, and effectively.

Understanding Bioidentical Estrogen

Lastly, if you need more estrogenic support for your body, I recommend the use of biochemically identical hormones. Biochemically identical hormones are molecularly identical to the hormones found in the human body. Moreover, they are produced in the laboratory from natural ingredients such as soy and wild yam, derived from plants, not horse urine. Since bioidentical hormones are biologically similar to the hormones your body produces, they do not appear to have the grave risks associated with conventional HRT.

The bioidentical estrogen that I typically recommend is estriol. Of the three types of estrogen produced within your body, estriol is the weakest and least potent. More importantly, several research studies have found that it is as effective as the stronger, more potent estrogens for treating menopause symptoms.

Not only is my program safe, gentle, and incredibly effective, but you can relieve menopausal symptoms, improve and support your health, and start feeling more like yourself again. The program also slows down the detoxification, breakdown, and elimination of estrogen, and safeguards you against postmenopausal conditions, such as osteoporosis and heart disease.

To summarize, my natural, healthy estrogen program consists of three options: (1) nutrients that have estrogen-like activity and can help to relieve symptoms of estrogen deficiency typically seen in menopause; (2) nutrients that can help you actually produce more of your own estrogen and also help to slow down your metabolism and excretion of the estrogen you do produce, thereby increasing yours to a higher and healthier level that can eliminate menopause symptoms and support your tissues and organs; and (3) biochemically identical estrogen replacement therapy.

Best of all, my program is very flexible. Simply take all of the information you'll find here and customize it to what feels best for your body. For example, some women love herbs, others don't. Some women like soy; others have trouble digesting it. By overlapping treatments from all the different options, you will be sure to find a combination that works best for you.

5

Benefit From Estrogen-Like Hormone Substitutes

There are many foods, herbs and nutrients that replicate estrogen's role in your body. I have found that a combination of plant-based foods and nutrients, yin herbs, and key vitamins are very helpful in combatting menopause symptoms in women who are estrogen deficient. These hormone substitutes provide a safe, estrogen-like effect. Using them in a combination that works best for you on a regular basis, in sufficient amounts, can improve your hormone status and greatly reduce menopause symptoms.

Estrogen Support with Phyto Foods

Flaxseeds

Essential fatty acids are critical for health and must be supplied daily by the diet, as the body cannot make them. The skin is full of fatty acids that, along with estrogen, provide moisture, softness, and smooth texture. When estrogen levels decline with menopause, moisture can continue to be provided to tissues of the skin, vagina, and bladder, as well as the hair, by increasing the intake of fatty acid–containing foods. Excellent sources of essential fatty acids are fish, nuts, and seeds, especially flaxseeds. Flaxseeds are particularly good for the skin and hair dryness that many women experience once they enter menopause.

Both ground whole flaxseeds, which are 30 percent oil by content, and cold-pressed organic flaxseed oil can be used as a food supplement, are excellent sources of the two essential oils, alpha-linolenic acid and linoleic acid. Flaxseed is unusual since it also contains a double source of plant-based estrogen. Both the oil and the flax lignan (a substance contained within the cellulose like material that provides structure to plants) contained within the seed have been researched for their weakly estrogenic effect.

A study published in the *British Medical Journal* described how shifting the diet toward phytoestrogen-containing foods can change certain menopause indicators. In this study, twenty-five menopausal women (average age: 59) were asked to supplement their normal diet with phytoestrogen-containing foods such as flaxseed oil and soy flour. The women consumed these foods over a six-week period. Smears from the vaginal wall were taken every two weeks to see if the addition of estrogen-containing plant foods would cause a beneficial hormonal effect on the vagina. Typically, the vaginal mucosa thins out and becomes more prone to trauma and infections as the estrogen level drops with menopause. Interestingly, the vaginal mucosa responded significantly to the additional ingestion of flaxseed oil and soy flour but returned to previous levels eight weeks after these foods were discontinued and the women went back to their usual diet.

Seeds and whole grains also contain lignans, which make up part of the structure of plants. Once plant lignans are eaten, intestinal bacteria convert them to substances that are weakly estrogenic and can provide additional nutritional support to menopausal women deficient in this hormone. This was confirmed in a study appearing in *Proceedings of the Society for Experimental Biology and Medicine*. Flaxseeds are 100 times richer in lignans than any other plant. Other sources of essential fatty acids include evening primrose oil, borage oil, and black currant oil. Unlike flaxseed oil, these other oils are not used as foods, but as nutritional supplements.

For women who are still having periods, flaxseed can act as a menstrual regulator. In a study conducted at the University of Minnesota, published in the *Journal of Clinical Endocrinology and Metabolism*, eighteen women with normal menstrual cycles ate normally for three cycles and then added 10 g of flaxseed powder per day to their diet for an additional three cycles. During the time that the women did not eat flaxseed, there were three cycles when no ovulation occurred. But when flaxseed was included, all of the women in the study ovulated every menstrual cycle. Thus, ground flaxseed was found to improve the estrogen-to-progesterone ratio favoring the levels of progesterone within the body. Progesterone production occurs only in ovulatory menstrual cycles.

Another very important benefit of ground flaxseed is that research studies have shown that it provides protection against breast cancer in women and, even, prostate cancer in men. Research studies in postmenopausal women with breast cancer found that flaxseed lignans reduce the growth and aggressiveness of the tumors and even enhance tumor death and destruction when fed muffins containing flaxseed. Women who were fed placebos- muffins without the flaxseed- did not show any of these benefits against breast cancer. Research studies have shown similar benefits on prostate cancer in men who have been diagnosed with this disease.

Our skin is filled with fatty acids that, along with estrogen, provide the moisture, softness, and smooth texture that we prize in beautiful and healthy looking skin. When our estrogen levels decline with menopause, we can continue to provide moisture to the skin, vagina, and bladder mucosa by increasing levels of essential fatty acid-containing foods. Flaxseed oil is particularly good for dry skin since it contains high levels of both fatty acids. In addition, fatty acids are a main structural component of all cell membranes and are found in high levels in such important tissues as the brain and nerve cells, adrenal gland, retina, and inner ear.

Besides relieving tissue dryness, the essential fatty acids found in flaxseed are needed by the body as precursors for the production of important hormone-like chemicals called prostaglandins. Body tissues manufacture over thirty types of prostaglandins. The proper balance of prostaglandins can play a major role in relieving and preventing many diseases that occur predominantly in the postmenopausal period.

For example, beneficial prostaglandins keep the platelets, a component of blood, from sticking or clumping together. This reduces the likelihood of heart attacks and strokes by preventing clotting of the blood and obstruction of the blood vessels. Since the incidence of heart attacks increases tenfold between the ages of fifty-five and sixty-five, this can benefit women who are in the postmenopausal period. In addition, they reduce inflammation, and thus the symptoms of arthritis. Many women date the onset of arthritis symptoms after menopause. Beneficial prostaglandins also stimulate immune function and helps insulin to function effectively.

Flaxseed oil is sold in opaque containers in the refrigerator section of most health food stores, as it is very sensitive to heat, light, and oxygen. Flaxseed oil bottles are dated to ensure that they are used quickly to preserve their freshness. Flaxseed oil can even be stored in the freezer, as can seeds and nuts, until you are ready to use them. It is also marketed as a ground meal and in capsule form.

I also recommend substituting flaxseed oil for butter. Flaxseed oil is the best substitute for butter that I've found. It is a rich, golden oil that looks and tastes quite a bit like butter. It is delicious on anything you'd normally top with butter—toast, rice, popcorn, steamed vegetables, or potatoes. Flaxseed oil is extremely high in essential fatty acids—the type of fat that is very healthy for a woman's body. Essential fatty acids improve vitality, enhance circulation, and help promote healthy hormonal function. Flaxseed oil is quite perishable, however, because it is sensitive to heat and light. For that reason, don't cook with it—cook the food first and add the flaxseed oil before serving. Also, keep it refrigerated even before opening it. Because flaxseed oil has so many health benefits, I highly recommend its use. You can find it in most health food stores.

Ground flax meal, which contains the whole seed, is also available in health food stores. It can be stirred into hot cereal like oatmeal or used in shakes and smoothies. It is an excellent source of fiber as well as phytoestrogens. Like flaxseed oil, it needs to be refrigerated to maintain its freshness. **I recommend taking 1 to 2 tablespoons of flaxseed oil each day or 2 to 4 tablespoons of ground flax meal.**

Pomegranate

Super fruits like pomegranate are a rich source of antioxidants like polyphenols, some of which have anti-inflammatory benefits. Pomgranates also contain a high content of anthocyanins which are a subcategory of plant bioflavonoids. These are the pigments that give these fruits their strong, beautiful colors like reds and purples and are also protective antioxidants.

In case you don't know what an antioxidant is, let me explain. An antioxidant is a substance that protects our bodies from free radical damage. A free radical is a type of oxygen molecule that freely moves inside cells, reacting with proteins, fats, and DNA, changing and damaging their structure and disrupting their functions. Free radicals are generated by the metabolism of oxygen and other chemicals, including cigarette smoke, unsaturated fats, food additives, and environmental chemicals—and even by aerobic exercise. Free radicals can cause an extreme amount of damage within our bodies.

Antioxidants help to protect us from free radical damage. Antioxidants unite with free radicals and deactivate them, preventing them from doing damage. A variety of substances have an antioxidant function, including vitamin C, vitamin A, beta-carotene, vitamin E, selenium, and glutathione. It is important to either include all of these antioxidants in the diet or take them as supplements.

There are also specific benefits for women in eating pomegranates. They contain natural plant estrogens which may be useful in relieving vaginal dryness, supporting bone health and balancing mood in menopausal women. According to a research published in *Cancer Prevention Research* and reported by the Cleveland Clinic, substances found in pomegranates may help prevent estrogen dependent breast cancers. Pomegranates contain polyphenols called ellagitannins that are converted to urolithin A and B in the intestines. These substances block an enzyme called aromatase that converts androgen (male hormones) to estrogen, which stimulates certain breast cancers.

Pomegranate has other health benefits. Early research on pomegranate juice suggests that it may improve blood flow to the heart is people with coronary heart disease as well as improve the lipid profile in diabetic patients. Research on kidney dialysis patients found that pomegranate juice reduced inflammation and kidney damage. According to research done at UCLA, it may also be beneficial in slowing the growth of prostate cancer. **I recommend taking 500 mg capsules of pomegranate extract, once or twice a day. You can also drink pomegranate juice which is less desirable because of its fruit sugar content.**

Soybean Isoflavones

Many research studies have confirmed that soybean-based products can actually help reduce and prevent menopause symptoms. Soybeans are filled with natural plant estrogens (or phytoestrogens) called isoflavones. Weak estrogenic activity is found in a variety of plant foods and herbs. However, for therapeutic purposes, only soybeans contain sufficient active compounds to approximate the effects of estrogen produced by the body. Soy contains two main phytoestrogens—genistein and daidzein, which belong to the class of chemicals called isoflavones.

Soy isoflavones were first discovered during the 1930s, but their potency was not assayed until the 1950s. At that time, genistein was found to be 50,000 times weaker than a powerful synthetic estrogen. Asian women eat much more soy products in their traditional diet than American women, whose isoflavone intake is virtually zero. This was confirmed in a study published in *The Lancet*, which found that Japanese women who regularly eat a range of soy products had 100 to 1,000 times more isoflavone breakdown products in their urine than Western women. Additionally, menopausal women in Japan are rarely troubled by symptoms such as hot flashes.

As weak estrogens, these compounds bind to estrogen receptors and act as a substitute form of estrogen in the body. They compete with the more potent estrogens made by a woman's body for these cell receptor sites. As a result, isoflavones can help to regulate estrogen levels.

High estrogen levels can worsen female problems like heavy menstrual flow, PMS, fibroid tumors of the uterus, endometriosis, and fibrocystic breast lumps. A soy-based diet can decrease the severity of these problems by reducing the toxic effects of the more potent estrogens made within our bodies on estrogen-sensitive tissues like the breast and uterus.

After menopause, when estrogen levels can become deficient, dietary sources of estrogen such as soy can provide much-needed hormonal support for the body. In fact, a diet high in isoflavone-rich soybeans can actually reduce the incidence of menopause symptoms. Asian women eat much more soy products in their traditional diet than American women, whose isoflavone intake is virtually zero.

In Japan only 10 to 15 percent of the women experience menopause symptoms. By contrast, 80 to 85 percent of women in the United States, Canada, and Europe who eat a traditional Western diet experience menopausal symptoms.

One study reported in the *British Medical Journal* examined how shifting the diet towards phytoestrogen-containing foods can change certain menopause indicators. In this study, 25 menopausal women (average age fifty-nine) were asked to supplement their normal diet with phytoestrogen containing foods like soy flour, flaxseed oil, and red clover sprouts. The women consumed these foods over a six-week period, each food for two weeks at a time.

Smears of the vaginal wall were taken every week to see if the addition of estrogen-containing plant foods would cause a beneficial hormonal effect on the vagina. (Typically, the vaginal mucosa thins out and becomes more prone to trauma and infections as the estrogen level drops with menopause.) Interestingly, the vaginal mucosa did respond significantly to the intake of soy flour and flaxseed oil (not to the red clover sprouts) but returned to its previous state eight weeks after these foods were discontinued and the women went back to their normal diets. Studies have also shown the benefit of soybeans in reducing hot flashes.

Other research studies have measured phytoestrogen excretion, comparing groups with a diet rich in soy and other phytoestrogens to groups eating the typical Western omnivorous diet. One study showed that men, women, and children in Japan and America who ate a diet high in soy foods like tofu, boiled soybeans, and miso excreted 100 to 1000 times more beneficial isoflavones in their urine than women in Finland and the United States who ate a meat and dairy based diet. In fact, isoflavone content tends to be 80 percent lower in the typical American or European meat- and dairy-based diet, than it is in a vegetarian-based diet.

Although this has been the subject of controversy, research studies are more aligned with the findings that isoflavones found in soybeans have the added benefit of being anticarcinogenic. Research has linked a high intake of soybean-based foods to the lower incidence of breast cancer and lower mortality from prostate cancer among Japanese women and men, respectively. Research studies done in the U.S. have confirmed the benefits of soy foods for prostate cancer. Other clinical studies have found that soy helps to lower cholesterol levels, thereby helping to reduce the incidence of heart attacks.

Soy is available in many forms in the United States. Tofu, an inexpensive, bland, curd-like soy product, can be found in most supermarkets and health food stores. Tofu will take on the flavor of any food that you cook it with, which makes it an ideal source of protein and essential fatty acids that you can add to soups, stir-fries, casseroles, and other dishes. Tempeh is a cultured soy product made of the whole soybean. Besides being a good source of protein, it contains vitamin B12, a nutrient needed for the production of healthy blood cells and nerve function. Purely vegetarian diets are often deficient in vitamin B12. Thus, adding tempeh can be helpful. Miso is often used to make a healthy, delicious soup.

One of the most interesting uses of soy is as a dairy substitute. Any product that comes from a cow is now available in a soy-based version. This includes soy milk cheese, sour cream, yogurt, cream cheese, and ice cream-like desserts. Although the soy cheeses generally tend not to be as tasty or textured as cow's milk based cheeses, they can still be used as good substitutes in recipes. Soy-based meat such as hot dogs, burgers, and other substitute meat products can be very delicious also. Be sure to look at the label of each product to make sure that it is not too high in either salt or fat.

Concerns about Soy's Side-Effects

It seems that we are bombarded on a daily basis with new information about soy—in some cases praising its benefits, and in other cases making it the scapegoat for everything from Alzheimer's to early maturation of teenage girls. While a handful of the critical studies have some merit, many are based on questionable research or test tube science. These studies really lose their impact when compared to the hundreds of clinical, animal, and epidemiological studies that attest to soy's health-protective benefits.

Still, I receive questions almost weekly about the dangers of soy and breast cancer and/or thyroid function. In my experience, I believe that it is probably safe for women with breast cancer to eat soy foods in moderation, with one caveat. In a study published in *Cancer Research*, researchers investigated the interactions between dietary genistein and tamoxifen and breast cancer by implanting estrogen-dependent breast cancer cells in mice who had had their ovaries and thymus removed. They found that genistein negated or overwhelmed the inhibitory effect of tamoxifen. Based on these findings, they urged postmenopausal women to exercise caution when consuming dietary genistein, found in soy foods or in supplements, while taking tamoxifen.

To date, I have not seen anything in the literature to negate this conclusion. Therefore, if you have breast cancer and are taking tamoxifen, I suggest that you use caution and avoid using pure soy isoflavones unless further, more conclusive studies contradict these findings. However, If you have questions about the advisability of using soy foods for your particular case, I recommend that you check with your doctor.

In the case of hypothyroidism, I believe that the concern over soy's impact on thyroid function is unwarranted. First, no well-controlled, statistically significant human studies have shown that soy interferes with thyroid function. In fact, several studies conducted on humans have found no difference in thyroid function between those women who ate soy and those who did not. Second, the lack of evidence surrounding this topic has led the FDA to reverse its earlier position that soy adversely affected the thyroid. Even more compelling is the fact that the American Foundation of Thyroid Patients has reviewed the current medical literature on soy and thyroid health and now recommends soy for all its members.

Based on the research as well as my experience, I see no reason for most women with a thyroid condition to avoid soy or soy products. The only exception I have made is for women who have inflammatory bowel disease and autoimmune thyroiditis, combined with a known allergy or sensitivity to soy. For this very small group of women, I recommend avoiding soy, as it may aggravate their condition.

Eating soy-based foods also has several other long-term health benefits. Unlike prescription estrogen, soy does not appear to have a carcinogenic effect on uterine cells or breast tissue. In fact, it appears to be cancer-protective for several reasons. Not only does soy reduce the production of estrogen within the body, but it also directly inhibits the growth of breast cancer cells. A review article appearing in the *Journal of the American Dietetics Association* noted that soybean intake is associated with reduced rates of prostate, colon, and breast cancer. Once again, we see this benefit in Japanese women, who have an incidence of breast cancer four to six times lower than that of women who do not include soy in their diet.

Other studies currently in progress suggest that soy can have a beneficial effect on both blood fats and bone metabolism. While estrogen is often prescribed to prevent heart disease and osteoporosis, soy offers a food-based approach to the same health issues.

Still, soy is not for everyone. Some women don't like the taste of soy foods and other women have difficulty digesting it. It is one option among many that you can choose from to help relieve menopause symptoms.

If you are allergic to soy, then obviously you need to avoid consuming it entirely. If you find that soy foods cause digestive upset such as gas, bloating, or intestinal discomfort, I suggest taking a high-potency digestive enzyme such as bromelain or papain whenever you consume soy foods, or simply opt for supplemental soy isoflavones capsules.

I recommend that you take in 50–100 mg of soy isoflavones each day, either through soy foods or isoflavone capsules, or a combination of both.

Isoflavones in Soy Foods

Whole soybeans (edamame) — 150 mg
Soy milk — 35–40 mg
Tempeh — 35 mg
Tofu — 35 mg

> ### Kathleen's Story
>
> When Kathleen first consulted with me, she had a busy career, lived on unhealthy but convenient fast food meals, and was 25 pounds overweight. She was postmenopausal, with high blood pressure and cholesterol. Moreover, she had lost considerable bone mass—even though she was only in her early 50s. She was very concerned about the negative direction that her health was going in and wanted to reverse this pattern.
>
> Kathleen was a perfect candidate for soy foods. She was delighted that she could substitute soy burgers for the high-fat, high-sodium cheeseburgers she had been eating, and started to explore other soy foods such as tofu, tempeh, soy milk, soy yogurt, and soy cheese. She also began adding healthy salads, soups, steamed vegetables, nuts, and other legumes to her diet. In addition to soy foods, I put Kathleen on a powerful program of nutritional supplements and bioidentical hormones.
>
> She was absolutely thrilled with the results—her excess weight fell off rapidly, her blood pressure and cholesterol dropped, and her bone mineral density improved. She enjoyed her new diet so much that she became increasingly interested in cooking and experimenting with healthy recipes—something she had never done before in her life!

The Healing Power of Plants

Many herbs are estrogen like in their activity, including common culinary herbs such as fennel and anise, as well as licorice. Other herbs, such as black cohosh and red clover, have been used medicinally as part of healing traditions for thousands of years. While their estrogenic activity is a small fraction of the activity of the estrogen a woman produces (at least 400 times less active), their benefit is that these herbs usually do not cause unwanted side effects for most women.

Black Cohosh

One of the most effective estrogen supportive herbs is black cohosh. Native to America, black cohosh was well known and accepted in Native American herbal medicine and was widely prescribed in colonial times as a treatment for menstrual cramps and menopausal symptoms.

The effectiveness and safety of black cohosh are well documented. Clinical studies have shown that black cohosh relieves hot flashes, night sweats, heart palpitations, headaches, and vaginal dryness and atrophy. It is also effective in relieving other symptoms such as depression, anxiety, sleep disturbances, and a decline in libido.

Currently, in Germany, a special extract of black cohosh is the most thoroughly studied and widely used natural alternative to hormone replacement therapy. This research has prompted at least six well-publicized studies on the standardized extract of black cohosh and its ability to treat menopausal symptoms. According to a review of five key studies on black cohosh from the *American Journal of Medicine*, black cohosh is most effective at easing hot flashes.

In one of the largest studies on black cohosh, women with menopausal complaints received 40 drops of liquid black cohosh extract twice a day for six to eight weeks. Within four weeks of treatment, a distinct improvement was seen in nearly 80 percent of the women. After six to eight weeks, all symptoms had completely disappeared in half of the women.

Another study found similar results. Scientists gave women with menopausal symptoms either high or low-dose black cohosh for a 12-week period. At the conclusion of the study, approximately 80 percent of both patients and physicians rated the treatment as "good to very good." The investigators reported no differences in either effectiveness or adverse reactions between the two groups.

Other studies have focused on black cohosh and its relationship to breast cancer. One in particular concluded that black cohosh actually inhibits the growth rate of breast cancer cells due to the herb's lack of estrogen-like effects in certain breast cancer cell lines whose growth is dependent upon estrogen. Laboratory experiments have shown that black cohosh inhibits the effects of estrogen-induced stimulation and actually binds to those receptors. By doing so, it does not increase production of endometrial cells, nor does it change the makeup of vaginal cells. Also, it does not exert estrogen-like effects on the endometrium or breast, nor does it exhibit any toxic, mutagenic, or carcinogenic properties.

Given its apparent safety, I consider black cohosh a safe therapy for women who suffer from the acute symptoms of menopause, such as hot flashes, night sweats, sleeplessness, vaginal dryness and mood swings. Klimadynon from BioNorica has shown to be an excellent source of black cohosh. Compelling research from several different journals, including *Maturitas: The European Menopause Journal* and *Menopause: The Journal of the North American Menopause Society*, has shown that Klimadynon (CR BNO 1055) safely and effectively eases hot flashes and night sweats, promotes plumping of the vaginal wall, decreases vaginal dryness, and even promoted bone growth. Moreover, Klimadynon did not cause proliferation of the uterine lining or of breast cells. This means that it, very likely, does not increase your risk of uterine or breast cancer.

Note: A study from the *Australian Adverse Drug Reactions Bulletin* found that, in rare instances, black cohosh can cause liver toxicity. More common and minor effects include occasional gastrointestinal disturbances, headaches, heaviness in the legs, and possible weight problems. There are no known drug interactions and the only contraindication is in pregnancy, with the possibility of premature birth due to overdose.

Additionally, an article in the *Journal of Agricultural & Food Chemistry* found that some three of 11 tested black cohosh supplements didn't even contain the herb! Instead, they contained less expensive extracts of a similar Chinese herb. To be sure this doesn't happen to you, I suggest buying black cohosh from a reputable retailer or look for BioNorica's Klimadynon brand.

To treat your menopausal symptoms safely and effectively, I suggest taking 40–80 mg of a standardized extract of black cohosh such as Klimadynon twice a day. This dose should contain 2 to 4 mg of the active components (triterpenes, calculated as 27-deoxyacteine). You should see results within four weeks. In my practice, I have seen women experience relief from hot flashes and mood swings in as little as two days to one week.

> ### Jennifer's Story
>
> Jennifer called me in a panic and said that she needed to come in and see me right away. Her menopause symptoms were making her feel so nervous and stressed that she felt shaky all the time, was unable to sleep because of her hot flashes or even concentrate well. She was on constant deadlines with her job and was terrified that she would be fired because she was having difficulty completing her assignments. As a single woman who was helping to support her own mother who was ill and bedridden, she could not afford to lose her income.
>
> When I saw Jennifer, she was distraught and obviously very worried. She was an attractive and nicely dressed woman but appeared pale and shaken. She did not want to take conventional HRT since she had had very uncomfortable side effects with oral contraceptives years earlier that made her feel bloated and anxious. She was concerned that conventional HRT would aggravate her current symptoms.
>
> I felt that Jennifer was an excellent candidate for black cohosh and recommended that she try this as an option, along with a high quality multi-nutrient supplement, additional vitamin E, vitamin C and bioflavonoids. I also recommended that she avoid all coffee, sugar, and alcohol, which could aggravate her nervousness, shakiness and hot flashes. She began the program immediately. I received a phone call from her within a few days, telling me that she was feeling much better, more calm and grounded and was able to work more effectively.

Red Clover

Red clover can also be useful for easing hot flashes and improving cardiovascular health. Red clover contains four phytoestrogens (estrogen-like plant compounds thought to have an effect on menopause-related symptoms such as hot flashes) called genistein, daidzein, biochanin, and formononetin, and has become increasingly popular among menopausal women here in the United States.

While some studies have questioned the efficacy of red clover, comparing it to that of a placebo, it does appear to help reduce hot flashes. According to a review of five studies published in *The American Journal of Medicine*, red clover helps to significantly reduce the frequency of hot flashes. Other research has shown that the herb is also beneficial for cardiovascular health. Both the aging process and menopause itself reduce the elasticity of major arteries (called arterial compliance). This tends to make blood vessels more rigid and less flexible. Over time, these changes can lead to high blood pressure, or hypertension, and increase the workload on the heart.

In one placebo-controlled study reported in the *Journal of Clinical Endocrinology and Metabolism*, red clover improved arterial compliance. Other known potential cardiovascular benefits of red clover isoflavones include the inhibition of platelet clumping or aggregation, which can clog arteries, and the herb's action as a potent antioxidant, which also helps reduce buildup of "bad" LDL cholesterol in arteries. **I recommend taking a standardized extract that contains 40 mg of total isoflavones.**

Restoring the Yin

Traditional Asian medicine maintains that health and well-being are believed to be a balance of two equally important, but opposing, principles—yin and yang. Yin is associated with attributes such as femininity, receptivity, calmness, coolness, and moisture. Yin also regulates the fluids, blood, and tissues of your body, as well as its structural components, including flesh, tendons, and bones. Yang, on the other hand, is associated with masculinity, aggression, heat, and dryness.

It also regulates your body's energy, which acts as the spark plug to your structural elements.

Balance between yin and yang is essential if you are to achieve and maintain optimal health and well-being. In younger, healthy women, the balance between this duality seems to be maintained almost effortlessly. Young women can become either very yin or very yang in response to the demands and stresses in their lives. They can study hard, work overtime, eat anything they want, and still have the ability to return to the balanced middle point, where yin and yang co-exist as a unified reality.

Maintaining an optimal yin-yang balance becomes much more difficult once you reach middle age and menopause, when it's common to experience symptoms such as hot flashes, night sweats, tissue dryness, insomnia, mood swings, and thinning of skin, hair, bones, and connective tissue. In the traditional Asian medical model, these symptoms occur, in part, because yin becomes deficient. To help bring your body back into balance, I suggest using a variety of yin herbs that work on the kidney network to improve blood and fluid circulation, ovarian health, and your sleep-wake cycle. In particular, I'd like to focus on royal jelly, dong quai, saffron, rosewater and geranium oil.

Royal Jelly

Royal jelly, the food of the queen bee, has been used for centuries to promote reproductive health and longevity and ease menopausal symptoms. Doctors from France have reported that women who ate royal jelly during menopause had a complete remission of symptoms, and some were even able to conceive again! Other doctors have found that royal jelly had a libido-increasing effect and helped promote vaginal secretions. Additionally, royal jelly has been found to be a natural antibiotic, fat metabolizer, immune booster, and metabolic catalyst, and even supports adrenal health.

I recommend using **1/4 teaspoon of the liquid form of organic royal jelly twice a day**. Additionally, women who are allergic to bees or have asthma should not take royal jelly. Be sure to avoid royal jelly from China. Recent reports have shown that royal jelly imported from this country has been found to contain trace amounts of a dangerous antibiotic called chloramphenicol. To avoid this concern, be sure to purchase royal jelly that is produced by bees from the United States under healthy, organic conditions. Royal jelly can be purchased at most health food stores or ordered from Glory Bee at glorybee.com or 800-456-7923. I like the Glory Bee products for my own personal use and have been using their products for many years!

Dong Quai

Dong quai is a Chinese herb (also called dang gui) that has been used for thousands of years as a female health tonic and to prevent or treat symptoms of PMS and menopause. Traditionally, dong quai has been used to treat abnormal menstruation and menopausal hot flashes. Many naturopathic physicians and herbalists today regularly prescribe this herb for their female patients.

In China, most women consume dong quai as a food, cooking the root in soup or other liquid mixture to soften it. **I recommend that you take dong quai in powdered form in a 500 mg capsule. Take two capsules two to three times a day.** Do not take dong quai if you are on a blood-thinner, as it may reinforce the effect of the anticoagulants and could increase your risk for bleeding.

Saffron

Saffron is a bright yellow Indian spice that is also used traditionally to reduce menopausal symptoms, enhance calmness, and diminish irritability. To preserve its medicinal properties, stir saffron into hot, cooked food. **Use 1/10 of a teaspoon or less per day**, as higher amounts can be toxic, causing stomach and intestinal maladies. Additionally, too much saffron can have a narcotic effect, causing sedation and sleepiness.

I also want to tell you about an amazing multi-herb blend called *Formula D-34*. This impressive blend of 10 herbs also works to restore kidney yin. In fact, a study of 20 menopausal women found that Formula D-34 significantly increased blood levels of estradiol, the most potent and chemically active estrogen produced by your body. Additionally, the women reported a considerable reduction in menopausal symptoms, including hot flashes, depression, and anxiety. Formula D-34 is made by Draco Natural Products. I have included this amazing formula as one of the components in my own hormonal support product that I formulated for women with estrogen deficiency.

Rosewater

Water infused with rose oil supports the yin and has a calming and cooling effect on the body. It is an excellent topical to **spray on the skin several times a day** if you are experiencing heat symptoms such as hot flashes, dry skin and hair, wrinkling, restless sleep, and insomnia. It helps to hydrate the skin and is gentle and non-irritating. It also acts as an anti-inflammatory and is soothing to irritated skin. Rosewater has a delightful, sweet scent.

Geranium Oil

This essential oil has a lovely, feminine scent and blends well with other essential oils. It supports the yin, which is very helpful for women in menopause, and has a calming, harmonizing effect on the mood and emotions. Many women describe its effect as relaxing and uplifting. It can be used by women of all ages, but is particularly helpful for women in menopause. Geranium essential oil can be added to bath water and is often incorporated into skin care products. It benefits the dry skin that affects many women in menopause and has also been used for inflammatory conditions like acne and eczema.

Vitamins that Reduce Menopause Symptoms

Like phytoestrogens found in plants and herbs, certain vitamins have also been found to offer a natural way to reduce the symptoms of menopause, such as hot flashes, night sweats, insomnia, headaches, nervousness, and irritability—with little risk of side effects. The two vitamins with the most research in the area of menopause are vitamin E and bioflavonoids.

Vitamin E

The original research on vitamin E's usefulness as an estrogen substitute was done between the 1930s and the early 1950s. Some of this research was done on breast and uterine cancer patients who were in menopause and were known to be poor candidates for estrogen replacement therapy, since it was understood as far back as the 1930's and 40's that estrogen could stimulate the growth of any remaining tumor cells.

Vitamin E was found to be both effective and safe in alleviating menopausal symptoms in these patients, and it could be safely used by breast cancer patients. Between 67 and 95 percent of the women followed in various studies had relief of such common menopausal symptoms as hot flashes, fatigue, mood swings, and muscle aches and pains. Vitamin E was less successful for the treatment of vaginal atrophy, being helpful in only 50 percent of the cases.

One such study from the *British Medical Journal* found that vitamin E not only helped reduce hot flashes in 64 percent of women tested, but also helped reduce symptoms of vaginal aging. Fifty percent of the women reported healing of vaginal atrophy, as well as a decrease in pain during sex.

A similar study published in the *Journal of the American Medical Association* found that of the 25 menopausal women treated with 10 mg of vitamin E, all found either complete relief or significant improvement in frequency and severity of hot flashes, as well as an improved mood and outlook on life. In another study of 66 women with menopause-related depression and irritability, 91 percent of the women found relief from their symptoms with vitamin E.

To relieve menopause-related symptoms, I suggest you take 400–1,600 IU of natural vitamin E daily, as d-alpha in a base of mixed tocopherols. Start with a lower dose and increase this by 400 IU every two weeks until the desired effect is achieved.

Oil-based capsules can also be used topically to treat irritation caused by the thinning of the vaginal walls that can occur at menopause. The capsule is opened and the vitamin oil applied directly to vaginal tissues. I recommend that women test the vitamin first to make sure that there is no skin reaction. A tiny amount of vitamin E can be applied over a few days before using larger doses topically.

Bioflavonoids

These substances are found in the peel and pulp of citrus fruits as well as in buckwheat. While bioflavonoids can be useful in helping relieve and prevent premenopausal symptoms, they can be equally useful for menopausal women. This is because bioflavonoids are a subclass of flavonoids called flavones which are weakly estrogenic. Happily, they can be used as a safe, nontoxic substitute for estrogen.

The potency of bioflavonoids is so low that they have no side effects for most women, yet they can relieve hot flashes as well as vaginal dryness. A study of ninety-four women at Loyola University Medical School showed the effectiveness of a bioflavonoids–vitamin C combination in controlling hot flashes for most of the women tested. In addition, bioflavonoids were used in this particular study as an estrogen substitute for cancer patients who cannot use traditional replacement therapy because their tumors are estrogen-sensitive. **I suggest taking 750–2,000 mg of bioflavonoids per day.** Bioflavonoids are considered to be very safe and have virtually no side effects.

6

Support Your Own Estrogen Production

You can also support hormone production in the central nervous system, ovaries, and adrenal glands, as well as reduce the breakdown and elimination of estrogen safely and gently with the use of specific nutrients. These can be used instead of or in addition to the hormone substitutes that I discussed in the previous chapter.

Because all hormone production begins in the brain, you can work to increase estrogen production through the brain or central nervous system. The hypothalamus is the master endocrine gland contained within your brain that regulates your production of sex hormones. This gland produces precursor hormones called gonadotropin releasing hormones (GnRH). When they are released, they travel to your anterior pituitary gland, where they stimulate the secretion of the follicle stimulating (FSH) and luteinizing hormones (LH). As you now know, these hormones then travel to the adrenals and ovaries, where they stimulate the production of estrogen, progesterone, and testosterone.

In order to keep the whole process working smoothly, FSH and LH need to be triggered by a balanced mixture of the key neurotransmitters necessary to produce these hormones. Neurotransmitters are naturally occurring chemicals that relay electrical messages between nerve cells throughout your body. The production of these vital chemicals is synthesized from certain amino acids, vitamins, and minerals that must be obtained through your diet or from supplementation.

For women who are in premenopause and are estrogen dominant, it is critical to increase levels of LH to help trigger ovulation and progesterone production. In the case of menopause and estrogen deficiency, just the opposite is true. You want to favor estrogen production. Additionally, you'll want to increase the neurotransmitter serotonin.

Serotonin

All neurotransmitters stimulate hormone production, but menopausal women are most in need of serotonin. Serotonin is an inhibitory neurotransmitter. This means it quiets down the processes of your body, rather than speeding them up. Within your brain, serotonin often inhibits the firing of neurons, which dampens many of your behaviors. In fact, serotonin acts as a kind of chemical restraint system.

Of all your body's chemicals, serotonin has one of the most widespread effects on the brain and physiology. It plays a key role in regulating temperature, blood pressure, blood clotting, immunity, pain, digestion, sleep, and biorhythms. It also produces a relaxing effect on your mood.

When you are low in serotonin, you are most likely not a lot of fun to be around. Low levels often lead to mood swings, depression, insomnia, chronic pain, food cravings, migraine headaches, and irritable bowel syndrome. It can even increase your likelihood of infection and sleep apnea.

Menopausal women are most at risk of decreased levels of serotonin, thanks to a complementary relationship between this neurotransmitter and estrogen. According to research from both the *American Journal of Psychiatry* and *Behavioral and Cognitive Neuroscience Reviews*, as goes estrogen, so goes serotonin. It appears that estrogen stimulates serotonin production. If you don't have adequate amounts of estrogen, you are not producing adequate amounts of serotonin. Additionally, low estrogen also triggers your brain to release monoamine oxidase (MAO), an enzyme that degrades serotonin. So decreased estrogen levels have a double-whammy effect on serotonin.

This relationship is the key to postmenopausal depression and anxiety. By increasing estrogen, you increase serotonin, and thereby elevate your mood and reduce many of the symptoms related to menopause.

The essential amino acid tryptophan is initially converted into an intermediary substance called 5-hydroxytryptophan (5-HTP), which is then converted into serotonin. While tryptophan is available as a supplement and is abundant in turkey, pumpkin seeds, and almonds, I've found that 5-HTP is a more effective and reliable option for boosting your neurotransmitter production. Numerous double-blind studies have shown that 5-HTP is as effective as many of the more common antidepressant drugs and is associated with fewer and much milder side effects. In addition to increasing serotonin levels, 5-HTP triggers an increase in endorphins and other neurotransmitters that are often low in cases of depression.

The Serotonin-Thyroid Connection

Serotonin is also intimately bound with thyroid hormone. Healthy thyroid function plays an important role in supporting healthy serotonin production and concentration, as well as preventing serotonin reuptake. As a result, strong, healthy thyroid levels result in an increased level of serotonin in the brain.

If you exhibit symptoms of low thyroid—cold hands and/or feet, weight gain, constipation, fatigue, dry skin, brittle nails, depression, loss of hair—then you need to have a thyroid test performed. If you are determined to have low or hypothyroid, I strongly suggest bringing your thyroid hormone up to normal levels to ensure that you have adequate, healthy levels of serotonin.

To maintain proper serotonin levels, it is helpful to take 100–200 mg of 5-HTP per day, preferably at bedtime. I recommend with all nutritional supplements, you should start at the lower to more moderate dosage (100 mg a day). Stay on this dosage for two weeks. If you don't notice a reduction in your symptoms, gradually increase the dosage by 50 mg every two weeks until you have either noticed a reduction in your symptoms or have reached the maximum dosage.

Serotonin also needs to be properly balanced with other neurotransmitters that have a more excitatory effect on the body and stimulate energy, zest for life, libido and a more rapid metabolism. If you naturally have a more placid, peaceful temperament and a tendency towards lower energy, weight gain, fluid retention, and even depression, stimulating the brain excitatory pathways that help to speed up the processes of your body will be more helpful for you.

The excitatory neurotransmitter pathways are primarily made up of substances like dopamine, norepinephrine, and epinephrine. Unlike serotonin, which has a calming and relaxing effect on your energy and behavior, excitatory neurotransmitters energize and elevate your mood. They act as powerful antidepressants and also support alertness, optimism, motivation, zest for life, and sex drive.

The excitatory neurotransmitters are derived from tyrosine, an amino acid produced from phenylalanine (another amino acid). A variety of vitamins and minerals, such as vitamin C, vitamin B6, and magnesium, act as cofactors and are necessary for the conversion of these amino acids into neurotransmitters.

To maintain optimum dopamine levels, take 500-1,000 mg of tyrosine per day. Be sure to take in divided doses, half in the morning and half in the afternoon. Do not take in the evening, as it may interfere with sleep.

Because creating a proper healthy balance between these two groups of neurotransmitters can be more challenging, I strongly advise that you undertake a program to properly balance your neurotransmitter levels under the care of a complementary physician or naturopath.

You should also have your neurotransmitter levels tested regularly. State-of-the-art neurotransmitter testing is currently available and can accurately pinpoint your exact levels of these essential brain chemicals. NeuroScience, Inc., (888-342-7272 or neurorelief.com) is a leader in the development of neurotransmitter testing. They have developed sensitive testing for these neurochemicals that can be done through your urine. The test is simple to do, non-invasive, and can be done in the privacy of your own home. In addition to NeuroScience, there are many other similar laboratories that offer neurotransmitter testing.

I would strongly recommend that you consider such testing if you suspect that you suffer from a moderate to severe neurotransmitter deficiency. Your health care provider will need to order these tests for you.

There are three key nutrients that will also help to raise estrogen levels — melatonin, glandulars, and ginseng through their effect on the brain and endocrine system. Let's take a look at each of them in more detail.

Melatonin

Melatonin is a hormone produced from serotonin and secreted by the pineal gland. Its secretion takes place at night and is inhibited by light. As such, it sets and regulates the timing of your body's natural circadian rhythms, such as waking and sleeping.

Unfortunately, as you get older, you produce less and less melatonin. This is due, in part, to menopause. Women who have poor sleep patterns, such as night shift workers, are also more likely to have decreased melatonin production.

As I mentioned earlier, melatonin is produced from serotonin, and serotonin production is stimulated by estrogen. Low estrogen equates to low serotonin, which results in low melatonin…which means you can't fall asleep or stay asleep easily.

In fact, a study from the *Annals of the New York Academy of Sciences* found that there is a cause-effect relationship between decreased nighttime levels of melatonin and the onset of menopause. Researchers found that women who took 3 mg of melatonin a day for six months enjoyed decreased FSH levels (with levels returning to those of a younger woman), and nearly a third of the menopausal women experienced a return of normal menstrual cycles. Even though estrogen and other hormone levels were not elevated during the study, a return of menstruation means more estrogen production. And, as I mentioned earlier, when women enter menopause, their levels of FSH and LH production in the pituitary increase in an effort to trigger greater estrogen production. Additionally, the study showed a significant improvement in thyroid function and relief of menopause-related depression in the women using melatonin.

Another research study published in the *Journal of Clinical Endocrinology and Metabolism* studied men and women over the age of 50 who suffered from insomnia to assess the best melatonin dosage necessary to promote healthy sleep. Researchers looked at three dosages: 0.1 mg; 0.3 mg; and 3.0 mg (the same dosage used in the *Annals of the New York Academy of Sciences* study). Unfortunately, they found that the 3.0 mg dosage had some downsides. It decreased body temperature and caused melatonin levels to stay elevated throughout the day. However, the lower doses—especially the 0.3 mg dosage—restored sleep without these negative side effects.

Research has also shown that melatonin is cancer-protective. One study looked at 250 patients with a wide variety of advanced, metastatic tumors, including lung cancer, breast cancer, gastrointestinal cancer, and head and neck cancer. None of the patients who received chemotherapy alone enjoyed a complete response, while six of the patients who received chemo and 20 mg of intravenous melatonin did, and another 36 patients achieved a partial response. Moreover, the one-year survival rate was significantly higher in the melatonin/chemo group (51 percent) than the chemo-alone group (23 percent). Researchers concluded that melatonin may be the secret weapon in the war on cancer.

To ensure that you have adequate levels of melatonin, I suggest supplementing with 0.3–1 mg at bedtime. Some women may find that they do better with a higher dosage. In this case, I suggest taking 1.5–3 mg. In my own hormone support product, I have erred on the side of caution and included 0.3 mg of melatonin. For melatonin to be effective, your bedroom should be dark, as light suppresses its release.

The following drugs deplete melatonin. If you are taking these drugs, be sure to supplement with adequate amounts of melatonin.

- Aspirin
- Ibuprofen
- Beta-blockers
- Calcium channel blockers
- Sleeping pills
- Tranquilizers

> ### *Carol's Story*
>
> Carol was a 68-year-old patient of mine who, for about 15 years after reaching menopause, experienced mild depression and mood swings. When she came to see me, her depression had worsened and sleeplessness had set in. Even more frustrating for her was that she felt sleepy and depressed during the day, but as soon as the sun went down, she became restless and couldn't sleep for more than three hours. This cycle of sleepiness and sleeplessness was beginning to affect her work and even her simple, everyday tasks, but even more upsetting, her marriage was starting to sour.
>
> Carol's situation is common in women who have neurotransmitter imbalances. Testing showed that Carol did indeed have a neurotransmitter imbalance—in particular, her serotonin levels were too low.
>
> I put Carol on a combination of melatonin, valerian root as well as other nutrients. Soon, she was feeling like her old self again and sleeping better than ever.

Glandulars

Glandular therapy involves the use of purified extracts from the secretory endocrine glands of animals. Most commonly, extracts are drawn from the thyroid and adrenal glands, as well as the thymus, pituitary, pancreas, and ovaries. Most extracts come from cows, with the exception of pancreatic glandular preparations usually drawn from sheep.

There are four common ways to extract glandulars. The first involves quick-freezing the material, washing it with a potent solvent to remove fatty tissues, distilling the solvent out, drying it, and then grinding it into a fine powder that is then encapsulated or pressed into tablets. The second mixes freshly crushed material with salt and water that also removes fatty tissues. It is then dried and ground into a fine powder to be placed in capsules or made into tablets.

In the third method, the glandular material is freeze-dried, then placed into a vacuum chamber to remove the water. It is then encapsulated. However, with this method, fatty tissues remain. The final method uses plant and animal enzymes to partially "digest" the material. It is then passed through a filter that separates out the fat-soluble molecules. The remaining material is then freeze-dried. This method seems to be quite effective. Due to the "pre-digestion," all biologically active substances remain intact and can be used therapeutically to support and restore your body's endocrine glands. Healthier endocrine glands are more likely to create healthier hormone production.

In the past, most experts believed that glandulars were not effective because the intestinal lining of a healthy person was impenetrable, and that proteins and large peptides could not breach its barrier. However, recent evidence has shown that large macromolecules can and do pass completely intact from the intestinal tract and into the bloodstream. In fact, there's further evidence to suggest that your body is able to determine which molecules it needs to absorb whole, and which can be broken down.

Both animal and human studies alike have proven this theory. In some cases, several whole proteins taken orally, including critical enzymes, have been shown to be absorbed intact into the bloodstream. Additionally, many smaller proteins and numerous hormones have also been found to be absorbed intact into the bloodstream, including thyroid, cortisone, and even insulin.

In essence, it means that the active properties of the glandulars stay active and intact, and are not destroyed in the digestive process. This is key to the success of glandular therapy, and explains why they clearly help to restore hormone function. When the gland is healthy, you de facto have fewer hormone-related problems because the feedback loop of the central nervous system and the endocrine glands are working properly. In essence, if you optimize the function, you bring all your hormones back into balance.

Examples of widely used and accepted glandulars involve the thyroid and the adrenals. Natural thyroid medications such as Armour Thyroid, Naturthyroid, and Bio-Thyroid have been the preference of complementary physicians for decades. Unlike many of the commonly prescribed brands of thyroid therapy that only replace a synthetic form of T4, these natural thyroid replacements contains the whole animal-derived thyroid gland, including T3 and T4. This is a significant difference. T3 is more physiologically active than T4, and is critical in regulating normal growth and energy metabolism. Without the use of glandulars, this type of natural thyroid replacement wouldn't be possible. However, the thyroid glandulars sold in the health food stores have the hormone removed and are used to support the function of your own gland.

Adrenal glandular preparations are even more common. With the stress epidemic in this country, the majority of Americans are walking around with major adrenal stress. Fortunately, whole adrenal extracts have been found to help restore the health and function of comprised adrenal glands. In one research study, eight women suffering from morning sickness (nausea and vomiting) who took oral adrenal cortex extract found relief within four days. A similar study gave both injected and oral adrenal cortex extract to 202 women also suffering from morning sickness. More than 85 percent of the women completely overcame their nausea and vomiting or showed significant improvement.

To support the endocrine glands that make estrogen (and other female hormones), as well as those that regulate estrogen production—including the pineal gland, which secretes melatonin—I suggest taking a good multi-glandular or single glandular product such as pineal or hypothalamus from a company like Standard Process. Standard Process is a leader in the field; however, the company does require a prescription from a health care practitioner. Other good products are also available in health food stores and should be used as part of a nutritional program to support your entire hormone system. I suggest consulting with a complementary health care provider if you are interested in using glandular therapy.

Ginseng

Panax ginseng is an ivy-like ground cover originating in the wild, damp woodlands of northern China and Korea. Its use in Chinese herbal medicine dates back more than 4,000 years. In colonial North America, ginseng was a major export product. The wild form is now rare, but panax ginseng is a widely cultivated plant.

Ginseng has a legendary status among herbs. While extravagant claims have been made about its many uses, scientific research has yielded inconsistent results in verifying its therapeutic properties. However, enough good research does exist to demonstrate ginseng's activity, especially when high-quality extracts, standardized for active components, are used.

Ginseng has a balancing, tonic effect on the systems and organs of the body involved in the stress response. It contains at least 13 different saponins, a class of chemicals found in many plants, especially legumes, which take their name from their ability to form a soap-like froth when shaken with water. These compounds (triterpene glycosides) are the most pharmaceutically active constituents of ginseng. Saponins benefit cardiovascular function, hormone production, immunity, and the central nervous system.

During times of stress, ginseng acts as a general stimulant, delaying the alarm phase in Selye's classic model of stress. The saponins in the ginseng act on the hypothalamus and pituitary glands, increasing the release of adrenocorticotrophin, or ACTH (a hormone produced by the pituitary that promotes the manufacture and secretion of adrenal hormones). As a result, ginseng increases the release of adrenal cortisone and other adrenal hormones, including estrogen, and prevents their depletion from stress. Other substances associated with the pituitary are also released, such as endorphins.

In a double-blind study published in *Drugs Under Experimental and Clinical Research*, two groups of volunteers suffering from fatigue due to physical or mental stress were given nutritional supplementation over a 12-week period. One hundred sixty-three volunteers were given a multivitamin and multimineral complex, and 338 volunteers received the same product plus a standardized Chinese ginseng extract. Once a month, the volunteers were asked to fill out a questionnaire during a scheduled visit with a physician. This questionnaire contained 11 questions that asked them to describe their current level of perceived physical energy, stamina, sense of well-being, libido, and quality of sleep.

While both groups experienced similar improvement in their quality of life by the second visit, the group using the ginseng extract almost doubled their improvement, based on their questionnaire responses, by the third and fourth visits. Thus, ginseng, when added to a multivitamin and multimineral complex, appears to improve many parameters of well-being in individuals experiencing significant physical and emotional stress. This is particularly important for women in menopause with diminished estrogen production.

Ginseng also enhances mental capacity, as demonstrated in both animal studies and clinical trials in humans. Improvements in logical deduction, reaction time, mental arithmetic, alertness, and accuracy have been observed. ACTH (the hormone that stimulates the adrenal cortex) and adrenal hormones, which ginseng stimulates, are known to bind to brain tissue, increasing mental activity and acuity during stress.

Many of my patients have used ginseng and have found it to have energizing effects. When trying to replace yin, I suggest using the more cooling Chinese and American forms of ginseng, and avoid Korean red ginseng, which is considered to be "hotter" and more yang. This type of ginseng can have the reverse effect, causing a decrease in normal menstrual flow and dryness of the skin and mucous membranes.

To further support hormone function at the central nervous system level, I suggest taking 100 mg of American or Chinese ginseng in capsule form twice a day. For maximum benefit, be sure to take a high-quality preparation, standardized for ginsenoside content and ratio. If this is too stimulating, especially before bedtime, take the second dose midafternoon, or take only the morning dose.

In addition to stimulating hormone production at the endocrine and nervous system levels, you can also use nutrients such as wheat germ oil and boron to increase estrogen production.

Nutrients that Increase Estrogen Production

Wheat Germ Oil

Wheat germ oil is rich in vitamin E, which we already know has mildly estrogenic properties. In fact, wheat germ oil contains the same fatty acids and other nutrients like vitamin E that your body needs to support and produce hormones such as estrogen.

Wheat germ oil is so effective, it has even been shown to increase estrogen production and reestablish healthy menstrual cycles in young women. Living under the stress of war is often associated with widespread disrupttion of menstrual cycles. This was true of women living in an internment camp in Manila during World War II. Doctors who treated these women observed that menstruation had stopped abruptly after the first bombing of Manila, before a nutritional deficiency would have been experienced. These physicians conducted a small study, published in the *Journal of the American Medical Association* (*JAMA*), in which 10 women with amenorrhea (a lack of menstruation) were given 20 drops of wheat germ oil as a source of vitamin E. The doses were taken orally, three times a day, for a period of 10 days, preceding the onset of each woman's expected menstrual flow. Of the 10 women, eight began to menstruate or had uterine bleeding.

Another study found that wheat germ oil was beneficial in treating vaginitis in menopausal women. One particular patient had such an extreme case of the condition that the physician couldn't even examine her. After 10 days on wheat germ oil, the burning eased and 17 days later, she reported to be "better than in months."

I have found wheat germ oil to be very effective in treating the entire range of menopausal symptoms, most notably hot flashes. I suggest taking 2,000–

2,400 mg of wheat germ oil in capsule form a day, in divided doses. I am fond of the Standard Process and Viobin brands (standardprocess.com and viobinusa.com).

Boron

Boron is a trace mineral found in such foods as apples, grapes, almonds, legumes, honey, and dark green leafy vegetables like kale and beet greens. According to a study conducted by the U.S. Department of Agriculture, there is some evidence that boron enhances estrogenic activity. When women on estrogen therapy supplemented their normally low-boron diet with 3 mg of boron, their blood levels of estrogen, specifically beta-estradiol, were significantly elevated. It appears that boron boosts estrogen production and mimics some effects of estrogen. There is also anecdotal evidence that boron may reduce hot flashes.

Moreover, boron is critical in the fight against osteoporosis. One study published in *Nutrition Today* found that boron reduced urinary excretion of calcium by 44 percent and significantly reduced excretion of magnesium as well. It also found that increased levels of both beta-estradiol and testosterone.

To help boost estrogen levels and prevent osteoporosis, I suggest taking 3 mg of boron a day.

Nutrients that Decrease the Breakdown and Elimination of Estrogen

While plant-based nutrients, vitamins, and minerals all work to support estrogen production, you can also decrease the metabolism and elimination of estrogen to help maintain higher levels of the hormone. This will also help to relieve symptoms of estrogen deficiency. Let's take a look at the best ways to accomplish this.

Women with estrogen dominance need to be sure they are breaking down, metabolizing, and eliminating excess estrogen effectively. However, women in estrogen deficiency need to do everything they can to slow down this breakdown and excretion cycle.

During estrogen metabolism in the liver, the most potent estrogen (estradiol) is converted into the mid-level potency form of estrone. They are both then metabolized to the weakest and least potent form—estriol.

Estrogen is also inactivated as it passes through the liver, where it is bound to sulfuric and glucuronic acid. This binding process inactivates the estrogen, inhibiting it from binding to tissues. It is then secreted into the bile and passed into the intestinal tract, where it is then eliminated from the body via bowel movements.

To slow this process down, you need hormone potentiators, nutrients that help to keep free estrogen from being reabsorbed by the body, thus elevating the level of estrogen circulating through the body. That's where PABA and cobalt chloride (or cobalt derived from vitamin B12) come in.

PABA

PABA (para-aminobenzoic acid) is a fat-soluble B vitamin necessary for the production of folic acid. It helps to break down protein in the body, support red blood cell production, and maintain the health of the intestines. PABA also works to absorb ultraviolet light, and may be useful in alleviating some skin conditions, such as the over-pigmentation or under-pigmentation of skin.

More importantly, studies indicate that PABA helps to safely and effectively impede the breakdown of estrogen and other hormones in the liver. Research has shown that higher levels of PABA are associated with better mood and outlook, less thinning hair, better vaginal lubrication, and increased libido—all of which are also indicative of higher estrogen levels. In fact, PABA is the only substance (other than testosterone) that has been proven to increase libido!

In addition to increasing estrogen levels, PABA has also been found to increase adrenal and thyroid hormone levels, as well as enhance the effects of cortisone. Because of its cortisone-like effects, PABA was used to treat rheumatoid arthritis in the 1940's. Specifically, PABA has been shown to be beneficial in helping to relieve the stiffness and pain associated with arthritis. In fact, high doses of PABA have been found to prevent and even reverse the accumulation of fibrous tissue.

One study from the *American Journal of Medical Sciences* found that rheumatoid arthritis sufferers who took a low doses of cortisone and high doses of PABA enjoyed considerable pain relief. Specifically, they found that patients who took 12 grams of PABA, along with low amounts of cortisone, enjoyed significantly more relief than those people taking cortisone alone.

Moreover, PABA has also been found to be effective in overcoming infertility. Researchers gave 16 infertile women 100 mg of PABA four times a day for three to seven months. Twelve of the 16 become pregnant.

If you are tired, depressed, irritable, or show signs of anxiety, you may be deficient in PABA. **I recommend taking 400 mg a day, which may be taken in divided dosages as a hormone potentiator. To reduce pain associated with arthritis, take 4–10 grams of PABA.**

Cobalt

One of the most exciting, and little known, nutrients for menopausal women is cobalt. Research has shown that cobalt slows down the excretion of estrogen, thus allowing you to better maintain your own production of estrogen, as well as that of supplemental estrogen.

Cobalt is able to retain estrogen and other hormones by stimulating production of heme oxidase. This, in turn, promotes the breakdown of cytochrome P450, a substance that normally metabolizes and detoxifies estrogen. By breaking down this substance, cobalt helps to prevent estrogen metabolism and excretion.

Physicians who have used cobalt have found that it has significant therapeutic benefits for their patients, helping to reduce night sweats, insomnia, hot flashes, depression, mood swings, and memory loss. It has even improved the therapeutic effects of women using conventional HRT who were not experiencing symptom relief due to their increased excreting of the hormones.

To impede the breakdown and excretion of estrogen, I suggest taking 400–500 mcg of cobalt a day. To further improve your cobalt status, you can also take 100–500 mcg of B12 a day. Research has shown that cobalt is supplied in your body by B12. If you have adequate amounts of B12, you are likely to have adequate amounts of cobalt as well.

7

Estriol - Your Body's Natural Estrogen

For women who want to use some type of hormone replacement therapy in addition to the natural therapies I've already discussed, there is a third option—estriol. Estriol is produced in the laboratory from active steroid molecules found in soy and wild yam. The resulting molecules are structurally the same as those produced in your body.

Of the three estrogens, estriol is the weakest, and more importantly, it is probably the safest type of natural estrogen. Based on various animal and human studies, it appears that estriol is less likely to promote excessive tissue growth, and even helps prevent breast and endometrial cancers.

Several human studies indicate that it may be the ratio of estriol to estradiol and estrone that is protective. Women with higher amounts of estriol in relation to the other hormones were less likely to develop cancer, perhaps because estriol attaches to estrogen receptors that might otherwise bind to much more potent forms of estrogen that more readily promote cell proliferation. And, unlike conventional HRT that may cause fluid retention, headaches, nausea, and the buildup of uterine tissue, estriol has few, if any, side effects.

One study published in the *Journal of the American Medical Association* found that estriol was particularly effective in treating vaginal atrophy, mood swings, and hot flashes. Researchers selected 52 symptomatic, postmenopausal women and separated them into four groups, giving each group either 2 mg, 4 mg, 6 mg, or 8 mg of estriol per day for six months. On average, women in every group experienced a decrease in their menopausal symptoms after one month of treatment. Furthermore, in three of the four groups, women who had ranked their symptoms as severe now felt that their symptoms were very mild.

Another study from *Alternative Medicine Review* found that estriol provides the protection of conventional HRT without the risks. Additionally, estriol was shown to ease menopausal symptoms, including hot flashes, insomnia, vaginal dryness, and urinary tract infections.

A study from Taiwan showed similar results. Researchers gave 20 menopausal patients, aged 44–62 years, 2 mg of estriol a day for two years. They found that estriol was significantly effective in easing menopausal symptoms (especially hot flashes and insomnia) in 86 percent of patients. Additionally, estriol did not cause proliferation of the uterine lining. This is great news for women at high risk for endometrial cancer, such as those who are significantly overweight.

Other studies have supported estriol's benefit in treating recurrent urinary tract infections. In a study from the *New England Journal of Medicine*, researchers looked at 93 postmenopausal women with a history of recurrent urinary tract infections. After four months of treatment, the patients using estriol needed to use significantly fewer antibiotics for their bladder infections during the course of the study. Additionally, 95 percent of those who received the estriol remained disease-free. The only side effects noted with the use of estriol have been occasional mild itching and irritation.

Early research also suggests estriol may offer some protection to your bones. One study in particular found that estriol significantly improved bone mineral density. Researchers divided 24 elderly women into two groups. The first group received 2 mg of estriol a day for six months, while the other received a placebo; both groups were given 1,000 mg of calcium chloride per day. They found the group who took estriol enjoyed an increase in bone mineral density, while the control group actually saw a decrease in bone density.

A similar study published in the *Journal of Obstetrics and Gynecology Research* found that menopausal women who received 2 mg of estriol a day for 50 weeks enjoyed a significantly slower breakdown of bone. This was most noticeable in women who had been in menopause for at least five years. Patients also reported an improvement in menopausal symptoms.

More importantly, researchers found that estriol did not stimulate the uterine lining, which translates to a reduced risk for uterine cancer. Plus, the fact that it attaches to estrogen receptors in your breast tissue means estriol may help to block the more potent, and therefore carcinogenic, estrogens like estradiol from attaching to these receptors.

Using Biochemically Identical Estrogen

Estriol can be taken orally or used topically. **If taken orally, I recommend using 2–4 mg daily, in capsule form. When used topically, I suggest applying one gram of the cream to your vagina every night for two to four weeks, then use twice a week for maintenance.** Many women with vaginal or bladder symptoms may choose just to use the vaginal cream locally, limiting their total body exposure to estrogen. However, I recommend covering the urethral and outer genital area with a thin layer of the cream as well as applying it intravaginally during the first few weeks of use.

In addition to estrogen alone, some researchers advocate the use of estriol in combination with estradiol (bi-estrogen or bivalent) or with estradiol and estrone (tri-estrogen or trivalent). In these combinations, the amount of estriol is far greater than the other forms of estrogen. In the case of trivalent estrogen, the ratios are usually 80 percent estriol and just 10 percent each estradiol and estrone. These combinations are also highly effective, and have also been shown to reduce menopausal symptoms, improve bone density, and increase "good" HDL cholesterol.

Estriol and all biochemically identical estrogen have to be prescribed by your physician. I have found that physicians in my area will often prescribe estriol when asked to by their patients. Estriol is available at most compounding pharmacies, as well as a few mainstream pharmacies. I recommend the Women's International Pharmacy in Madison, Wisconsin, which sends estriol formulations to physicians throughout the U.S. You can find them online at womensinternational.com or by calling 800-279-5708.

8

Estrogen Breakdown and Elimination from the Body

In the previous chapters, I've discussed a number of foods, herbs, plants, vitamins, minerals, and even neurotransmitters all work to help you produce and maintain vital, healthy levels of estrogen. I've also shared with you information about bioidentical estrogen replacement therapy.

In this chapter, I discuss safeguards, so that any estrogen, whether it's your own or estrogen derived from HRT, is handled by your body in the safest, least toxic way. This will greatly reduce your risk of diseases that can accompany menopause, including breast cancer, heart disease, and arthritis, as well as help to significantly improve your overall health and well-being.

While estrogen is being produced or supplemented in the body, it also needs to be broken down (metabolized) and excreted. Otherwise, our estrogen levels would rise to unhealthy levels that can cause health problems due to estrogen excess. Our body's solution to keeping estrogen levels healthy and balanced is to breakdown or metabolize estrogen in the liver and then secrete it into the digestive tract where it is further changed and then eliminated through the digestive tract and kidneys. This should occur as a healthy cycle of production, breakdown, and excretion.

During this process, estrogen circulates in the blood throughout your body and passes through your liver. Your liver then metabolizes it from its more potent forms, estradiol and estrone, to a more chemically inactive and safer form, estriol. When the liver is healthy, this occurs efficiently. The estrogen metabolites are then secreted into the bile and, from there, into your digestive tract.

There are several substances that help to facilitate this process. These include B vitamins, DIM, calcium d-glucarate, d-limonene, fiber, and probiotics.

Vitamin B Complex

The vitamin B complex is a group of 11 separate, water-soluble nutrients: B1 (thiamine), B2 (riboflavin), B3 (niacin), B5 (pantothenic acid), B6, B12, biotin, folic acid, para-aminobenzoic acid (PABA), choline and inositol. In addition to regulating mood and restoring energy, B vitamins have been shown to help your liver inactivate estrogen.

The B complex vitamins specifically have been shown to help your liver breakdown your more potent estrogens into the weaker, but effective, estriol. Estriol is the least potent and safest form of estrogen, yet when present in sufficient levels; it is very effective in ameliorating and eliminating many symptoms of estrogen deficiency, such as hot flashes, vaginal dryness, and urinary tract conditions.

PABA, which I discussed earlier, also has a protective benefit, as it slows down the metabolism of many hormones, including estrogen. This helps to promote a healthier overall hormone balance

Additionally, like magnesium, B vitamins also help convert essential fatty acids taken in through your diet into inflammation fighting prostaglandins. This anti-inflammatory effect helps relieve inflammatory conditions that become more prevalent after menopause like rheumatoid arthritis, Sjogren's syndrome and other serious health issues.

To help promote the healthy breakdown of estrogen into estriol, I suggest taking 50–100 mg of a vitamin B-complex a day. Be sure it includes 50–100 mg of vitamin B6 and 400–500 mg of PABA.

DIM

Diindolylmethane, or DIM, is a plant-compound found in Brassica veggies such as broccoli, bok choy, cauliflower, cabbage, and Brussels sprouts. Researchers have found that this compound is quite beneficial in promoting estrogen metabolism. This is because DIM helps to metabolize estrogen into its safer form.

During estrogen metabolism, the most potent form of estrogen (estradiol) is converted into estrone. Estrone then becomes either 2-hydroxyestrone, a "good" estrogen metabolite, or 16-alpha-hydroxyestrone--a "bad" estrogen metabolite. The good metabolite (2-hydroxyestrone) is then converted into 2-methoxyestrone and 2-methoxyestrodial.

This is where DIM comes in. Research has shown that when DIM is ingested, it not only encourages its own metabolism, but that of estrogen. While it is not an estrogen or even an estrogen-mimic, its metabolic pathway exactly coincides with the metabolic pathway of estrogen. When these pathways intersect, DIM favorably adjusts the estrogen metabolic pathways by simultaneously increasing the good estrogen metabolites and decreasing the bad 16-alpha-hydroxyestrone.

The research confirms this action. In a study from *Epidemiology*, American researchers took urine samples from 34 healthy postmenopausal women. They then added 10 grams of broccoli a day to the women's diets. After taking another urine sample, researchers found that this dietary change significantly increased the 2-hydroxyestrone to 16- alpha-hydroxyestrone ratio.

Supplementing with DIM may also be protective against breast cancer. Since higher levels of bad estrogen circulating in the bloodstream have been associated with higher breast cancer rates, scientists theorized that by increasing the good to bad estrogen ratio, you could protect against estrogen dependent cancer.

In a study published in 1998, researchers in England looked at estrogen pathways to determine if in fact the ratio of the good 2-hydroxyestrone to the bad 16-alpha-hydroxyestrone actually affected breast cancer risk. They took urine samples from more than 5,000 women age 35 years and older. These samples were then frozen and stored for up to 19 years. Researchers found that those women with the highest good estrogen metabolite to bad estrogen metabolite ratio had a 30 percent decreased risk for breast cancer.

A similar study looked at the dietary habits of postmenopausal Swedish women aged 50 to 74. When asked how often, on average, they consumed a wide variety of foods, including 19 different commonly eaten fruits and vegetables, researchers found that those women who ate 1 to 2 servings of Brassica foods a day had a 20 to 40 percent lower risk of breast cancer than those women who ate virtually none.

Finally, a study from *Biochemical Pharmacology* found that DIM may have another intriguing benefit. Researchers at the University of California at Berkeley found that DIM not only blocked DNA synthesis in human breast cancer cells, but also stopped the cells from spreading. They discovered that DIM also caused the cancerous cells to die. I am very excited about this early in vitro research.

In the United States, researchers collected and tested the urine of nearly 11,000 women aged 35 to 69. At the time of testing, all women were cancer-free and not on HRT. After an average storage time of 5.5 years, the samples were tested for 2-hydroxyestrone and 16-alpha-hydroxyestrone levels and compared to those women who had developed breast cancer in that time. Researchers found that the women who had higher ratio of 2-hydroxyestrone to 16-alpha-hydroxyestrone at the start of the study were at less risk for breast cancer.

Once researchers became more confident that the 2-hydroxyestrone to 16-alpha-hydroxyestrone ratio was a good predictor of breast cancer risk, they set out to determine if consumption of *Brassica* vegetables such as broccoli and cabbage could influence this ratio. In a study from *Epidemiology*, American researchers took urine samples from 34 healthy postmenopausal women. They then added 10 grams of broccoli a day to the women's diets. After taking another urine sample, researchers found that this dietary change significantly increased the 2-hydroxyestrone to 16-alpha-hydroxyestrone ratio.

A similar study looked at the dietary habits of postmenopausal Swedish women aged 50 to 74. When asked how often, on average, they consumed a wide variety of foods, including 19 different commonly eaten fruits and vegetables, researchers found that those women who ate 1 to 2 servings of Brassica foods a day had a 20 to 40 percent lower risk of breast cancer than those women who ate virtually none.

Finally, a study from *Biochemical Pharmacology* found that DIM may have another intriguing benefit. Researchers at the University of California at Berkeley found that DIM not only blocked DNA synthesis in human breast cancer cells, but also stopped the cells from spreading. As mentioned earlier they discovered that DIM also caused the cancerous cells to die.

In addition to eating more Brassica vegetables like broccoli and cauliflower, I recommend taking 30 mg of DIM a day with meals.

D-Glucarate

Glucuronidation, a detoxification process that occurs in the liver, depends on glucuronic acid, a chemical produced within the body which is similar to calcium d-glucarate, a naturally occurring substance found in many fruits and vegetables. As estrogen circulates through the blood, it passes through the liver, where it is bound to glucuronic acid. This binding process inactivates the estrogen, inhibiting it from binding to tissues. It is then secreted into the bile and passed into the intestinal tract, where it is then eliminated from the body via bowel movements.

Unfortunately, certain bacteria in the intestinal tract secrete an enzyme called betaglucuronidase (B-glucuronidase) which can sabotage the glucuronidation process. B-glucuronidase breaks the newly formed estrogen-glucuronic acid bond apart, which reactivates the estrogen. This free estrogen can then be reabsorbed by the body, thus elevating the level of estrogen circulating through the body.

Luckily, eating a diet rich in glucarate or using glucarate supplements helps to decrease the level of B-glucuronidase by allowing the bond between glucuronic acid and estrogen to be maintained so the body can rid itself of excess estrogen. This helps to prevent your own level of estrogen from rising to toxic levels.

To reduce the total amount of circulating estrogen, I recommend taking 500 to 1,000 mg of glucarate per day with meals. This supplement is very well tolerated with no toxicity or known drug interactions.

Glucarate-Rich Foods

Apples	Brussels sprouts
Apricots	Cherries
Broccoli	Lettuce

Limonene

Another ally to help lower your total estrogen load is limonene, a compound usually found in citrus fruits, especially lemons and oranges. In addition to supporting glucuronidation, limonene also promotes healthy detoxification. Specifically, it has been shown to help prevent the development of estrogen-dependent breast cancer by stimulating detoxification enzymes in the liver.

A study published in *Cancer Research* tested to see if limonene could reduce or regress breast cancer in rats. Researchers fed a limonene-rich diet to rats that had developed breast tumors. They found that the rats that were given this diet had significant tumor shrinkage as compared to the control group. However, when the limonene was discontinued, the tumors reappeared. Additionally, researchers found that limonene inhibited the spread or metastasis of the cancer.

To help reduce free-floating estrogen in your body, I recommend taking 500-1,000 mg of limonene per day or every other day. Note: Women who are allergic to citrus should not take limonene. Additionally, while it appears to be safe and without toxicity, pregnant or nursing should not take limonene since no research has been performed that specifically examines its effect on fetal development.

Limonene-Rich Foods

Caraway	Oranges
Cherries	Mint
Dill	Tomatoes
Lemons	

Fiber

Dietary fiber is a key component to eliminating excess estrogen from your body. Once estrogen is broken down and neutralized by your liver, it is secreted into your bile. From there, it enters your small intestines. In your intestinal tract, fiber works by binding to estrogen and removing it through bowel movements. According to a study from Tufts University Medical School, vegetarian women excrete two to three times more estrogen in their bowel movements than do other women who eat a diet lower in fiber and higher in fat. This is great news for estrogen dominant women who are trying to reduce the estrogen load in their body.

In addition to regulating estrogen levels, fiber also binds to cholesterol. This helps to keep your bad cholesterol levels in a healthy range.

Plus, fiber is key for preventing constipation, colon cancer, and many other intestinal disorders. (More than 85,000 cases of colon cancer are diagnosed each year.) Once ingested, fiber undergoes bacterial fermentation in the colon. This process produces butyrate, the main energy source for colonic epithelial cells, which are needed for a healthy, cancer-free colon. This effect was verified in a study published in the *Scandinavian Journal of Gastroenterology*. Researchers followed the health of 20 patients who had undergone surgical treatment for colon cancer. The volunteers were given fiber in the form of psyllium seeds. After one month of supplementation, fecal concentration of butyrate increased by 47 percent.

There are two types of fiber: soluble and insoluble. Soluble fibers (dissolvable in water) are found in fruits, vegetables, nuts, and beans. Insoluble fibers (not dissolvable in water) are found in oatmeal, oat bran, sesame seeds, and dried beans. Sadly, the refining process has removed most of the natural fiber from our foods, creating a nation of people grossly lacking in fiber.

To ensure that you are getting adequate amounts of both kinds of fiber (and therefore ensuring the effective elimination of excess estrogen), be sure to eat whole-grain cereals and flours; brown rice; all kinds of bran; fruits such as apricots, prunes, and apples; nuts and seeds; beans, lentils, and peas; and a wide variety of vegetables. Several of these foods should be included in every meal. Moreover, when you eat apples and potatoes, enjoy them with their skins.

You can further supplement your diet with fibers like oat bran and/or psyllium (1-2 tablespoons per day, mixed with 8-12 ounces of water and swallowed immediately after stirring). You may also try guar gum (which is helpful in regulating your blood sugar level) and pectin (which is derived from apples and grapefruit and can lower the amount of fat that you absorb from your diet). Simply combine 1/2 teaspoon guar gum and 500 mg of pectin with 8-12 ounces of water. Stir and drink immediately. Use one to three times a day.

Probiotics

High intake of saturated fats, commonly found in foods such as dairy, butter, and red meat stimulate the growth of unhealthy, anaerobic bacteria in the intestinal tract. These bacteria chemically change the breakdown products of estrogen into forms that can be reabsorbed back into the body. These bacteria split estrogen from the binding substances that inactivate it in your liver. This splitting process causes free estrogen to be reformed within your intestinal tract. As this free estrogen is reabsorbed into the circulation, it increases free estrogen levels within the blood.

To suppress the growth of these unhealthy bacteria, I suggest that you not only reduce your intake of saturated fat (which can lead to the problem in the first place), but that you also use probiotic supplements. Probiotics help to recolonize your intestinal tract with healthy bacteria such as L. acidolphilus and B. longum. **I recommend taking probiotics that contain at least 1-3 billion live, healthy organisms per day.**

Part III:
How Healthy Lifestyle Supports Estrogen Levels

9

How Diet Affects Your Estrogen Levels

The quality of your lifestyle also plays a very important role in determining the level of estrogen in your body as well as the severity of your menopause symptoms. Choosing to eat a healthy diet, managing your level of stress and engaging in a regular exercise program will go a long way towards assuring a symptom free menopause. I discuss the role of healthy lifestyle and estrogen in this chapter.

Diet plays a very important role in determining the health of menopausal women. The foods you choose may trigger hot flashes and other unpleasant menopausal symptoms, as well as increase your risk of developing such serious diseases as heart attacks, strokes, cancer, and arthritis. On the other hand, foods chosen wisely for their high nutrient content and easy digestibility can decrease and even prevent symptoms of menopause.

The traditional American diet tends to work against us, because it is laden with unhealthy fat, sugar, salt and stimulants. If you follow this diet without making modifications as your body ages, your health will suffer. To change your eating habits in ways that will help create optimal health and well-being during your menopausal years requires knowledge about important concepts of nutrition, much of which never gets applied to the lives of many women in menopause.

This chapter contains essential information about diet that you may use to change your own habits toward optimal health. I have used these guidelines with my patients and they have been delighted with the beneficial results. The first section discusses the foods that you should emphasize for good health. In the second section, I will provide information on which foods to avoid or limit.

Foods That Ease Menopausal Symptoms

This type of diet includes high-nutrient foods such as beans and peas (legumes), whole grains, foods containing essential and healthy oils (including raw seeds and nuts), certain fish, and lots of fresh fruits and vegetables. There is evidence that this dietary approach can help relieve and prevent symptoms of menopause. These types of foods predominate in the traditional diets of many Asian and African cultures. Interestingly, menopausal symptoms tend to be much less prevalent and severe in these cultures. For example, these symptoms occur in 10 to 15 percent of Japanese women at midlife, in contrast with 80 to 85 percent of American women. Diet is thought to play a major role in the different ways women experience menopausal symptoms. Let us look at the benefits each of the healthy foods can bring you during your midlife years.

Beans and Peas (Legumes)

Soybean-based products actually help reduce and prevent menopausal symptoms. Soybeans are loaded with natural plant or phytoestrogens, called isoflavones. The estrogen-like isoflavones, particularly genistein and daidzein, were identified decades ago by researchers. Large quantities of soybeans are consumed in the traditional Japanese diet, providing as much as 30 to 100 mg of isoflavones per day. This may be one reason that the women report fewer menopausal problems.

As weak estrogens, these compounds bind to estrogen receptors and act as a substitute form of estrogen in the body. Although menopausal women are deficient in estrogen, the isoflavones can help reduce common symptoms, such as hot flashes and vaginal dryness. In addition, foods containing isoflavone may also have an anticarcinogenic effect, which could explain the lower incidence of breast cancer among Japanese women and lower mortality from prostate cancer among Japanese men.

U.S. studies have confirmed the benefits of a soy-rich diet in reducing the risk of breast cancer. For example, a study reported in the *American Journal of Epidemiology* found that women who had the highest consumption of legumes were 54 percent less likely to develop uterine cancer.

Dietary studies show that men, women and children in Japan, as well as Americans following a macrobiotic diet or vegetarian diet, excrete 100 to 1000 times more isoflavones in their urine than people in Finland and the United States who eat a meat- and dairy-based diet, which has an isoflavone content 80 percent lower than a vegetarian-based diet.

A study published in *The British Medical Journal* described how shifting the diet towards phytoestrogen-containing foods can change certain menopause indicators. In this study, 25 menopausal women (average age of 59) supplemented their normal diet with phytoestrogen-containing foods such as soy flour, flaxseed oil, and red clover sprouts over a six-week period. Smears from the vaginal wall were taken every two weeks to see if the addition of estrogen-containing plant foods would cause a beneficial hormonal effect on the vagina. Typically, the vaginal mucosa thins out and becomes more prone to trauma and infections with menopause. Interestingly, the vaginal mucosa responded positively to the ingestion of soy flour and flax oil, but returned to previous levels eight weeks after these foods were discontinued.

Another study involved eighty postmenopausal women who are were given either soy (with premeasured phytoestrogen content) or Premarin (the most frequently prescribed form of estrogen in the United States). Both the soy and estrogen ERT were found to have beneficial effects on both blood fats and bone metabolism. Soy isoflavones are currently available in capsule or powder forms as nutritional supplements. Optimally, a woman should ingest from 30 to 60 mg per day.

Legumes in general are excellent foods for menopausal women. Common sources include garbanzo beans, kidney beans, lima beans, black beans and lentils. All legumes are an excellent source of protein. When combined with whole grains, the two foods provide the full range of essential amino acids, the building blocks of protein.

In addition, legumes are an excellent source of fiber. This enables their nutrients, such as protein and carbohydrates, to be absorbed more slowly. This has many health benefits. The slow digestion of legume-based carbohydrates can help regulate the blood sugar level. As a result, legumes are an excellent food for women with blood sugar imbalances or diabetes. The fiber can help normalize bowel function and lower cholesterol levels by promoting excretion of cholesterol through the bowel movements.

Legumes are excellent sources of many other nutrients needed by menopausal women. These include calcium and magnesium, which are essential for strong bones and healthy muscle tone. Legumes also contain high levels of potassium, which help regulate the heartbeat as well as provide muscle tone. Legumes are very high in iron, copper and zinc. Sufficient iron intake is particularly important for women with heavy menstrual bleeding who are beginning menopause. Legumes are also high in vitamin B-complex, essential for healthy liver function. The liver metabolizes estrogen so that it can be excreted efficiently from the body.

Whole Grains

Healthy grains for menopausal women include oats, corn, barley, millet, buckwheat, wild rice, brown rice, and whole wheat. As with legumes, many whole grains are an excellent source of phytoestrogens. Whole grains contain lignans, a material that is used to form the plant cell wall. Lignans, like isoflavones, are weakly estrogenic and can provide additional nutritional support to menopausal women deficient in this hormone.

In addition, certain grain like plants such as buckwheat, are good sources of another flavonoid called rutin. This flavonoid is particularly helpful in its ability to strengthen capillaries and reduce heavy menstrual bleeding when women are just entering menopause. Flavonoids, like rutin, along with vitamin C, have been used in medical studies to reduce heavy bleeding during this time, and for bleeding due to fibroid tumors and spontaneous abortions. One study of women who miscarried multiple pregnancies concluded that the bioflavonoid-vitamin C combination allowed 78 percent of high-risk women studied to carry their pregnancies to full term.

The high fiber content of whole grains also helps regulate estrogen levels because of the ability of fiber to bind estrogen in the intestinal tract and remove it from the body through bowel movements. As described earlier, estrogen circulates in the blood throughout the body, including the liver. The liver metabolizes estrogen from its more potent forms, estradiol and estrone, to a chemically inactive and weaker form, estriol. When the liver is functioning in a healthy manner, this occurs efficiently. The estrogen metabolites are then secreted into the bile and from there into the digestive tract. This whole process is called the enterohepatic circulation of estrogen.

A high-fat, low-fiber diet promotes the growth of certain bacteria in the intestinal tract that act chemically on these estrogen products. These bacteria convert the estrogen products back to estrone and estradiol, allowing reabsorption of the estrogen back into the body. As mentioned earlier in this book, estrone is the primary type of estrogen produced by the body after menopause, and estradiol is the type of estrogen produced by the ovary during the active reproductive years.

As a result of the intestinal bacteria, the levels of these two estrogens rise higher than estriol, their primary breakdown product. This abundance of the more potent forms of estrogen may not present a healthy estrogen profile. Research studies have shown that estradiol and estrone, as the more chemically active and potent forms of estrogen, may predispose women toward developing breast cancer, while estriol, a much weaker form of estrogen, may confer protection against breast cancer. Thus, a high-fiber, low-fat diet may help regulate not only the estrogen levels, but the types of estrogen circulating through a woman's body. A number of studies have shown that vegetarian women excrete two to three times more estrogen in their bowel movements than do women eating the typical high-fat, low-fiber diet.

Besides regulating estrogen levels, the high-fiber content of whole grains binds to cholesterol, increasing its excretion from the body through the digestive tract. This helps lower blood cholesterol levels, reducing a significant risk factor for heart attacks in postmenopausal women. The fiber in grain is very helpful in relieving constipation, as well as preventing other diseases of the digestive tract such as diverticulitis and hiatus hernia. Fiber may also have a protective effect against developing colon cancer, a disease also found more commonly in people who eat a high-fat, low-fiber diet.

Whole grains are excellent sources of carbohydrates capable of stabilizing blood sugar and helping eliminate sugar craving. They help prevent or control diabetes mellitus, a dangerous disease that predisposes people toward heart disease, blood vessel problems, infections and blindness. Fifty percent of our population over age 60 have blood sugar abnormalities, due in great part to the tremendous amount of high-sugared foods and sweets Americans eat. Whole grains, with their natural sweetness, can satisfy much of this craving in a healthful way.

In addition, whole grains are a major source of complete protein when combined in a meal with legumes. Whole grains also contain many excellent nutrients for menopausal women. They contain high levels of vitamin B and vitamin E, both of which are critical for healthy hormonal balance and regulating estrogen levels. This occurs through their beneficial effect on both the liver and ovaries. Whole grains' vitamin B and vitamin E content also help combat the fatigue and depression that can occur with the onset of menopause. Grains are high in magnesium which helps reduce muscle tension. They are also high in calcium, necessary for healthy bones and to relax muscle tension. Finally, whole grains are high in potassium. Potassium has a diuretic effect on body tissues and helps reduce bloating, which can be a problem for postmenopausal women.

Essential Fatty Acid-Containing Foods

Healthy essential oils are extremely beneficial for menopausal women. Linoleic acid, which belongs to the Omega-6 family of fatty acids, is primarily found in raw seeds and nuts. Good sources include flaxseed, pumpkin seeds, sesame seeds, sunflower seeds, and walnuts. The other essential fatty acids are members of the Omega-3 family and are primarily found in certain fish such as trout, salmon, mackerel, as well as some plant sources like flaxseeds, soy, pumpkin seeds, walnuts, and green leafy vegetables. Both essential fatty acids must be derived from dietary sources because they cannot be produced by the body.

The body does not primarily burn the essential fatty acids for energy, unlike the saturated fats found in red meat, eggs, dairy products, and a few plants such as palm oil. Instead, these fatty acids have special functions in the body necessary for good health and survival. The skin is full of fatty acids that, along with estrogen, provide moisture, softness and smooth texture. When the estrogen levels decline with menopause, moisture continues to be provided to the skin, vagina and bladder mucosa by increasing levels of fatty acid-containing foods. Flaxseed oil is particularly good for dry skin because it contains high levels of both fatty acids. In addition, fatty acids are a main structural component of all cell membranes and are found in high levels in such important tissues as the brain and nerve cells, retina of the eye, adrenal glands and inner ear.

Besides relieving tissue dryness, essential fatty acids are also needed by the body as precursors for the production of important hormone-like chemicals called prostaglandins. There are over 30 types of prostaglandins manufactured by tissues throughout the body. The proper balance of prostaglandins can play a major role in relieving and preventing many diseases that occur predominantly in the postmenopausal period.

The series one prostaglandins are manufactured by the body from linoleic acid. These prostaglandins have many beneficial effects. One member of the series, called prostaglandin E, or PGE, is particularly helpful for menopausal women. It relaxes the blood vessels and improves circulation. It keeps the platelets, a component of blood, from sticking or clumping together. This reduces the likelihood of heart attacks and strokes by preventing blood clotting and obstruction of the blood vessels. Since the incidence of heart attacks increases ten-fold between the ages of 55 and 65, PGE can benefit women greatly. In addition, PGE prevents inflammation, reducing the symptoms of arthritis. For many women, arthritis symptoms begin after they go through menopause. PGE also stimulates the immune system and helps insulin function effectively.

The series 3 prostaglandins are manufactured from the eicosapentaenoic acid (EPA) found in fish such as salmon and trout. They are also produced more slowly from plant sources containing alpha-linolenic acid. As mentioned earlier, flax oil is a particularly good food source of alpha-linolenic acid. One member of this series called PGE 3 has anticlotting effects similar to those of PGE. They also help reduce the likelihood of heart attacks and strokes when manufactured by the body in high levels. PGE 3 also decreases triglycerides levels, another risk factor for heart attacks.

It also helps prevent the manufacture of PGE 2, an undesirable prostaglandin made from arachidonic acid, a fatty acid derived primarily from dietary sources of red meat and dairy products. Unlike PGE and PGE 3, arachidonic acid-derived PGE 2 actually promotes platelet aggregation or clumping, thereby initiating potentially dangerous clot formation. It also causes inflammation and fluid retention, which can predispose postmenopausal women towards arthritis and high blood pressure. Thus, it is important to favor fish, seeds, and nuts as sources of protein to promote production of the "good" prostaglandins.

Vegetables

Vegetables are excellent foods that come in a wide variety of flavors, colors and textures. They are important for health because they are extremely rich in many vitamins and minerals. Recent research in the past two decades has also emphasized their importance in protecting postmenopausal women from diseases such as heart attacks, strokes, cancer, and immune system breakdown.

Vegetables high in vitamin A usually have an orange, red, or dark green color. These include squash, sweet potatoes, pepper, carrots, kale, and lettuce, as well as many other common foods. Unlike animal-based sources of vitamin A, which contain an oil-soluble form of this vitamin, plant sources contain a precursor form of vitamin A called beta carotene. Beta carotene is converted to vitamin A by the liver and intestines once ingested into the body. This form tends to be very safe and is found in high doses in many foods. For example, one glass of carrot juice or a sweet potato each contains 20,000 international units [IU] of beta carotene. Many people eat two to three times this amount in their daily diet.

Research shows that vitamin A will protect against cancer and immune system deficiency. Of particular interest to menopausal women are studies showing that vitamin A may protect against breast cancer. Other research studies suggest that a high intake of plant foods containing beta carotene protects against heart attacks in high-risk people.

Many vegetables are also high in vitamin C, which has a protective effect against heart attack, cancer, and immune system problems. Vitamin C is particularly important for transitional menopausal women because, along with iron and bioflavonoids, it can protect against excessive menopausal bleeding. Research studies also suggest that vitamin C may help protect women from developing cervical cancer as well as vitamin A does. Vitamin C is important for wound healing and healthy skin. Vegetables high in vitamin C include potatoes, pepper, peas, tomatoes, broccoli, brussels sprouts, cabbage, cauliflower, kale and parsley.

Vegetables contain many other important nutrients such as iron, magnesium, and calcium that protect against osteoporosis, anemia and excessive menstrual bleeding. Leafy green vegetables, such as beet greens, collards, and dandelion greens, are excellent sources of these important nutrients. Other vegetables also have health enhancing properties. Onions and garlic decrease the blood's clotting tendency and lower serum cholesterol, which can help decrease the incidence of stroke and heart attack. Studies indicate that ginger root, onions, and mushrooms may have a similar effect. Certain mushrooms may even stimulate immune system function. Some vegetables such as kelp are high in iodine and trace minerals, essential for healthy thyroid function. Use kelp as a seasoning to sprinkle on vegetables and grains. Finally, vegetable fiber contributes to healthy bowl function and regulates levels of cholesterol and estrogen. It also promotes more efficient excretion of fat and estrogen through the intestinal tract. Be sure to eat your vegetables raw or lightly steamed to preserve their nutrient value. Do not boil or overcook vegetables, because vitamins and minerals can be lost through improper preparation.

Fruit

Fruits are an exceptional source of bioflavonoids and vitamin C which helps to control excessive menstrual flow as well as provide the body with weak plant sources of estrogen. The inner peel and pulp of the citrus fruit is an excellent source of bioflavonoids and, in fact, is used for commercial production of bioflavonoid supplements. This is, unfortunately, the more bitter part of the fruit that many women discard, unaware of the health benefits the inner peel and pulp can provide. Also, the skin of grapes, cherries and many berries are rich sources of bioflavonoids. So, it is better to eat the whole fruit rather than just drink the juice.

Adequate potassium intake is necessary for good health, and fruits are very good food sources of potassium. Potassium helps lower high blood pressure and protects against heart disease; it also decreases bloating and fluid retention. Medical studies show that potassium is beneficial in reducing menopause-related fatigue. Fruits high in potassium include bananas, oranges, grapefruits, berries, peaches, apricots and melons. Fruits are also an excellent source of vitamin C, which provides important protection against cancer and infectious diseases as well as heart disease. Most whole fruits contain some vitamin C—berries, oranges, and melons provide exceptionally high levels of this essential nutrient. Yellow and orange-colored fruits such as papaya, persimmon, apricot and tangerine should be included in your diet because of their high vitamin C content.

Although fruit is high in sugar, the high fiber content of the whole fruit slows down digestion, curbs appetite and stabilizes the blood sugar level. The high fiber content of many fruits make them excellent foods for women who experience constipation. A recent study published in the *Journal of the National Cancer Institute*, also found that a high intake of fruits and vegetables appears to confer some protection against developing breast cancer. This is because fiber seems to reduce levels of circulating estrogens by binding to estrogens in the intestines and promoting their excretion from the body through the bowel movements. Pineapple and papaya also contain enzymes that help to break down protein, so they promote food digestive function and speed up bowel transit time.

Be aware that fruit juice does not contain the bulk or fiber of whole fruit, so it does not stabilize blood sugar or have beneficial effects on bowel function. Juice acts more like the simple sugars found in candy, so it should be used sparingly. The whole fruit retains the sweet flavor and makes a healthy substitute for candies, cookies, cakes and other highly sugared foods. Use it as a snack or dessert instead of cookies, candies, pastries or ice cream.

Foods to Avoid or Limit with Menopause

On the other hand, diet can have a negative effect on your health as you go through and beyond menopause, if your food selection is poorly chosen. Foods described in this section either accentuate menopausal symptoms or add to the risk of developing diseases that increase in incidence during the postmenopausal period. These include heart disease, stroke, high blood pressure, cancer, arthritis and diabetes, to name only the most common ones.

Caffeine-containing Foods

Caffeine-containing foods include beverages such as coffee, black tea, cola drinks, and chocolate. These foods are used almost universally in our culture, both as stimulants and as emotional "treats." Caffeine belongs to a class of chemicals called methylxanthines, central nervous stimulants that increase alertness and energy level. Many menopausal women use a caffeinated beverage on a regular basis to combat fatigue and provide a pick-up in the morning. This practice may accelerate during menopause when fatigue is often worse due to poor sleep quality. Hot flashes and perspiration can recur throughout the night, leaving women depleted of energy and exhausted.

Unfortunately, there are many negatives to the use of caffeinated beverages. Caffeinated beverages can actually be a trigger for hot flashes. Caffeinated foods and beverages such as coffee, black tea, cola drinks and chocolate can trigger hot flashes because they tend to dilate the small blood vessels. Spicy food or hot drinks may have the same effect.

Caffeine is an addictive chemical and a person often requires large amounts to provide wakefulness and alertness. Regular caffeine users who stop caffeine intake abruptly may experience withdrawal symptoms such as headaches, mood changes, and increased fatigue. Psychological symptoms such as anxiety, irritability and mood swings due to hormonal deficiency are increased with caffeine intake.

In addition, caffeine has a diuretic effect and increases the loss of many essential minerals and vitamins such as potassium, zinc, magnesium, vitamin B and vitamin C accelerates with caffeine intake. Coffee also reduces the absorption of iron and calcium from food and supplemental sources, particularly when used at mealtimes. Several studies have confirmed caffeine as a significant contributor to osteoporosis. Discussed in a 1997 review article in the *Family Practice News*, this research found that consumption of more than three cups of coffee per day tripled the risk of hip fractures in susceptible women and also increased the risk of spinal fractures. Finally, caffeine use is linked to an increased incidence of nodules and tenderness in women with benign breast disease.

Postmenopausal women at high risk for a heart attack or stroke because of family tendency or blood fat profile may want to avoid caffeine. Caffeine increases blood cholesterol and triglyceride levels, which are risk factors for heart attacks. In addition, caffeine raises the blood pressure, another risk factor for heart attacks and strokes (hypertension becomes increasingly prevalent with age). Caffeine also causes the heart to beat faster and increases the excitability of the system that conducts electrical impulses through the heart. This can lead to irregular heartbeats in susceptible women.

Luckily, many substitutes are available for women who like either the taste of coffee or the pick-me-up that it produces. Water processed decaffeinated coffee is often the easiest substitute to start with for women who like the flavor of coffee. Coffee substitutes that are grain-based, such as Postum and Cafix, are even better and ginger tea can also have a vitalizing and energetic effect.

Alcohol

Alcohol will intensify almost every type of menopausal symptom. As a result, I recommend that women with active symptoms limit their intake or avoid alcoholic beverages entirely. The list of symptoms of menopause affected by alcohol intake includes hot flashes and mood swings. In fact, alcohol is a major trigger for hot flashes. Unlike caffeine, alcohol is a central nervous system depressant, so its intake can increase menopausal fatigue and depression. This is particularly pronounced in women with night sweats and insomnia whose sleep quality is already poor.

In addition, alcohol has a diuretic effect on the body. During our active reproductive years, estrogen helps keep the skin and other tissues plump by causing fluid and salt retention in the body. As our estrogen levels begin to wane, excessive intake of alcohol can further dehydrate the skin and tissues, including the vaginal and bladder mucosa. Alcohol's diuretic effect also causes the loss of excessive amounts of essential minerals through the urinary tract. These include minerals needed for healthy bones such as calcium, magnesium and zinc. Alcohol is also a contributor to osteoporosis. An article in the *Family Practice News* reviewed several studies on osteoporosis, which found that women who consumed more than seven ounces of alcohol per week nearly tripled their risk of hip fracture.

Alcohol also irritates the liver. It is metabolized by the liver to a chemical called acetaldehyde, which is liver toxic. In addition, excessive alcohol cannot be metabolized to glucose or glycogen (the storage form of glucose). Instead, it is metabolized and stored in the liver as fat. Excessive fat deposition in the liver can eventually lead to scarring and cirrhosis. Excessive alcohol intake can also affect the liver's ability to metabolize estrogen and can elevate the body's blood estrogen levels, particularly of the more chemically active forms of estrogen.

On the positive side, alcohol in small amounts can be a pleasurable social beverage. When used in amounts not exceeding four ounces of wine, ten ounces of beer, or one ounce of hard liquor per day, it can have a pleasant, relaxing effect. It makes us more sociable and enhances the taste of food.

Small amounts of alcohol may also increase the high-density lipoproteins, a type of blood fat that protects people against heart attacks. However, for optimal health, I recommend using alcohol no more than once or twice a week; this is true for women in midlife with no obvious menopausal symptoms.

Sugar

Sugar is one of the most overused foods in the United States. It is primarily utilized as a sweetening agent in the form of sucrose, which most of us know as white, granular table sugar. Sugar is a main ingredient of cookies, cakes, soft drinks, candies, ice cream, cereals and many other foods. Many women are unaware of how prevalent it is in convenience foods such as salad dressings, catsup, relish, and even some prepackaged main courses in the supermarket. Foods sold in natural food stores are highly sugared, too, although with different types of sweeteners such as fructose, maple syrup and honey. As a result of this national sweet tooth, the average American eats more than 120 pounds of sugar per year.

This dietary sugar is eventually metabolized to its simplest form in the body called glucose. Glucose by itself is essential for all cellular processes, because it is the major source of fuel our cells use to generate energy. However, when the body is flooded with too much sugar, it becomes overwhelmed, cannot process the sugar effectively and overreacts by pumping out large amounts of insulin. This is the hormone that helps drive glucose into the cells where it can be used as energy. When too much insulin is secreted, the blood sugar level falls, and hypoglycemia can occur. With continued overuse of sugar, the pancreas eventually "wears out" and is no longer able to clear sugar from the blood circulation efficiently. The blood sugar level rises and diabetes mellitus is the result. This tendency toward diabetes or high blood sugar levels increases dramatically after menopause. Research studies show that more than 50 percent of Americans have blood sugar imbalances by age 65.

Excess sugar intake also depletes the body's reserve of B-complex vitamins and many essential minerals by increasing their rate of utilization and sugar metabolism. This can increase anxiety, irritability and nervous tension that many women feel as they move into menopause. One research study even suggests that a diet high in sugar may impair liver function and affect the liver's ability to metabolize estrogen. Highly sugared foods also promote tooth decay and gum disease. Many women, however, are addicted to sugar and have a difficult time controlling their intake once they start eating sugary foods.

Because sugar is so deleterious to good health, menopausal women might consider avoiding sugar entirely or limiting its use to small amounts on social occasions. Sugar can be easily substituted in recipes by using fruit, sugar substitutes like stevia, brown rice syrup, or smaller amounts of more concentrated sweeteners. Also, become a label reader. If canned and bottled foods such as salad dressings, soft drinks, or baked beans have sugar near the top of the list, the product probably contains too much sugar. Search out alternatives that don't contain sugar or items using it in very small amounts. If you crave sweets, keep fresh or dried fruits handy such as apples, bananas or dried figs. Whole fruit should satisfy your craving for sweets and has the added benefit of being high in many essential nutrients.

Salt

Condiments and food additives such as table salt and monosodium glutamate (MSG) generally contain large amounts of sodium. Sodium is one of the body's major minerals. Primarily found in the body's extracellular compartment in conjunction with potassium, the primary intracellular mineral, sodium helps regulate water balance in the cells. Water tends to accumulate where sodium is prevalent. Thus, an overabundance of sodium relative to the body's potassium levels can lead to edema, bloating and sometimes high blood pressure. These problems are very common in menopausal women who are increasingly at risk for developing cardiovascular problems with age. In addition, fluid retention often adds to the excess pounds that can be so irksome to women after menopause. Many women complain that they gain 10 to 15 pounds after menopause and that the weight is very difficult to lose, even with dieting and exercise. Of even greater concern is the fact that excess sodium is a risk factor for osteoporosis because it accelerates calcium loss from the body.

Unfortunately, as with sugar, salt is prevalent in the American diet. In fact, salt and sugar are often found together in large amounts in frozen and canned foods, cheeses, potato chips, hamburgers, hot dogs, cured meats, pizzas and other common foods. Many of us eat so much salt (far beyond the recommended 2000 mg or 1 teaspoon per day) that our palates have become jaded. Many people feel that food tastes too bland without the addition of salt.

Luckily, many other available seasoning options are much better for your health. For flavoring, use garlic, basil, oregano and other herbs. Fresh foods such as vegetables, grains, legumes, and meat contain all the salt we need, so added table salt isn't necessary. As for sugar, read the labels before you buy bottled, canned or frozen food. Don't buy a product if salt is listed as a main ingredient (near the top of the list). Many brands in the health food stores and supermarkets now distribute foods labeled "no salt added" or "reduced salt content." Be sure to buy these rather than the high-salt content foods. Also, eat plenty of fresh fruits and vegetables because they are excellent sources of potassium and other essential nutrients. Potassium helps balance the sodium in the body and regulates the blood pressure to keep it at normal levels.

Red Meat, Dairy Products and Saturated Oils

At first glance, it may not be apparent that red meat, dairy products and saturated oils have much in common. However, they are the main sources of fat in the typical American diet. Unlike the healthy fats that were described in the preceding section (found primarily in vegetable sources such as raw seeds and nuts, leafy green vegetables and fish), these fats are derived from saturated fat sources. When used in excess, they contribute to such common health problems as heart disease, cancer, obesity and arthritis. Unfortunately, 40 percent (rather than the ideal 20-25 percent) of the calories in the American diet come from unhealthy, red meat-derived saturated fats.

Saturated fat tends to increase the cholesterol levels in the blood, particularly the high-risk, low-density lipoproteins that initiate the plaque formation in the blood vessels. Plaque formation can eventually lead to heart attacks and strokes. In contrast, the "good" fats derived from fish and vegetable sources can prevent heart attacks by reducing the tendency for the blood to clot. A high-saturated fat diet can also lead to obesity in women of all ages. Menopausal women are particularly at risk because their metabolism slows down with age and they burn calories less efficiently. One gram of fat contains nine calories versus the four calories contained in one gram of protein or carbohydrate. As a result, fatty foods are much higher in calories per unit weight. Although saturated fats do provide the body with a concentrated source of energy, very few of us need these extra calories. Instead of burning the fat for energy, we tend to store it in our cells as excess poundage.

As mentioned earlier, a high-fat, low-fiber diet is also associated with colon cancer, prostate cancer in men, and some breast cancer in women. In a study published in the *Journal of the National Cancer Institute*, 2,300 volunteers were examined as to their dietary habits with emphasis on their fat and oil intake. Women with breast cancer were found to have diets high in animal fats. Women who consumed olive oil on a daily basis had a significantly lower incidence of breast cancer.

One theory concerning the correlation between saturated fat and the risk of breast cancer is that a high-fat diet promotes the conversion of estrogen metabolites by anaerobic bacteria in the intestinal tract to forms of estrogen that can be easily reabsorbed back into the body. This elevates the blood estrogen level with the types of estrogen that may increase the susceptibility to breast cancer in certain women. In contrast, lowering the amount of dietary fat, while increasing the amount of high fiber foods in the diet, can help reduce the risk of hormone-dependent cancers in women.

Many American women base their meals on red meat and dairy entrees like steaks, chops, oversized meat sandwiches, and cheese sandwiches. Unfortunately, large amounts of red meat-based protein can increase the risk of osteoporosis. Red meat protein is acidic; when a woman eats red meat in excessive amounts, her body must buffer the acid load that red meat creates. One way the body accomplishes this is by dissolving the bones. The calcium and other minerals released from the bones help restore the body's acid-alkaline balance. (This process does not occur with dairy products, which already contain calcium.)

One study comparing the incidence of osteoporosis in meat-eating women (omnivores) with that in vegetarians found a dramatic difference in bone density after age 60. Between the ages of 60 and 89, vegetarian women lost 18 percent of their bone mass, but meat-eating women lost 35 percent of their bone mass—quite a striking difference. Other studies show that the amount of protein eaten will make a difference in actual calcium levels; protein intake over three ounces a day causes loss of the calcium from the urinary tract. This has been found to be true even in low-risk groups such as young, healthy males.

Finally, red meat, dairy products, and saturated oils (such as palm-kernel oil) are difficult to digest. As women age, they secrete less hydrochloric acid and fewer of the digestive enzymes needed for fat and protein breakdown in the intestinal tract. In one study, 40 percent of postmenopausal women lacked hydrochloric acid. Without sufficient hydrochloric acid, meat and other sources of protein are difficult to break down and thus, cannot be utilized properly by the body. In addition, calcium and iron absorption becomes more difficult without sufficient stomach acid.

Women who are concerned about eliminating dairy products from their diet because dairy foods are great sources of calcium can choose many other good food sources of calcium. These include nondairy milk substitutes such as almond and soy milks, beans and peas, raw seeds and nuts, green leafy vegetables, and canned salmon. Using a daily calcium supplement is probably a good idea because you are assured of receiving an optimal amount of calcium.

For optimal protein intake, your diet should emphasize whole grains, beans and peas, seeds, nuts and fish high in the beneficial omega-3 fatty acids. It is best to eliminate red meat and dairy products or use them occasionally in small portions. A truly optimal diet for the postmenopausal woman is one with high-nutrient content, low-stress foods and easy digestibility.

Summary Chart:

Foods for Menopause Relief
Beans and peas (legumes)
Whole grains
Essential fats
Raw seeds and nuts
Green leafy vegetables
Fish
Vegetables
Fruits

Foods to Limit or Avoid
Caffeine-containing foods
Coffee
Black tea
Cola drinks
Chocolate
Alcohol
Sugar
Salt
Red meat
Dairy products
Saturated oils

10

Managing Stress for Healthy Estrogen Levels

I have yet to meet a woman who does not struggle with stress. In fact, 10 percent of the American population—between 20 and 30 million people—exhibit clinical signs of stress and anxiety each year, and another 10 percent struggle with depression severe enough to warrant medication. Women of all ages, from preadolescence to post-menopause, are affected by stress, anxiety, and depression, with no one age group more affected by stress than another. And I can promise you that I have had my share throughout the years. Unfortunately, there is no way to eliminate it completely.

But the hectic pace at which many of us live our lives exhausts our adrenal glands and nervous systems and lowers our resistance to disease. Given all that, it's no wonder that stress often impedes a woman's ability to function optimally with co-workers, friends, and family.

What is Stress?

Stress is defined as a demand on physical or mental energy, as well as the distress this demand causes. Stress can be emotional, psychological, social, chemical, and/or physical in origin. It can be acute and sudden, as when a car cuts in front of you on the freeway. There are also persistent, chronic forms of stress, such as loneliness or the demands of raising children or caring for an aging parent. Changing jobs, getting a parking ticket, meeting new people, going away on vacation, competing in a tennis match, or giving a speech can all cause stress.

What you perceive as stress is purely subjective. A situation that one person considers manageable, another person may see as dangerous or threatening. People's perception of stress depends on their attitude toward challenges and change, their emotional and psychological coping skills, and their physical capability to respond to stress and recover quickly.

Unfortunately, millions of people lack the ability to effectively handle stress. As a result, we often trigger an output of chemicals within our bodies meant to help cope with stress. These chemicals have a profound effect on our physiology, affecting how we breathe, how blood circulates throughout the body, and even our level of muscular tension. If these stress chemicals are triggered only occasionally, the body does not suffer physical damage from their release. However, when triggered repeatedly, these chemicals may exhaust the body, causing unpleasant symptoms and, eventually, physical breakdown and disease.

Specific physical symptoms of stress include fatigue, insomnia, shortness of breath, heart palpitations, sweating, light-headedness, a craving for sweets, alternating constipation and diarrhea, low blood pressure, and blood sugar disturbances. Emotional signs of stress include anxiety, nervousness, and mood swings.

Stress-related symptoms may occasionally be so intense that they can interfere with a person's ability to function. For example, anxiety disorders such as claustrophobia (fear of closed or narrow spaces) and agoraphobia (fear of open or public places) may actually cause affected individuals to avoid social and work situations that can trigger their fears. I have had patients who reported having panic episodes when driving their car on a freeway or when presenting a speech before a large audience. If this sounds like you, believe me, you are not alone. Nearly 10 percent of the U.S. population—that's 20 to 30 million people—experience phobias, panic attacks, and other anxiety disorders in any given year.

Stress and Our Bodies

Whether your stress is triggered by a crazy commute, a busy household, an angry spouse or child, a demanding job, a difficult neighbor or family member, or even a poor self-image and too much self-criticism (which are very common issues for most of us), every woman has a point where the strain and anxiety start to take their toll. The problem is many women don't hear the warning messages their bodies send out—partly because they're too stressed out to listen, and partly because they don't know what the messages are.

Most women know that irritability, loss of sleep, appetite changes, tense muscles, and a tendency to catch whatever "bug" is going around can be signs of stress. But did you know that excessive stress can increase your risk of developing infectious diseases, including genital herpes and bladder infections? Researchers have even seen a relationship between stress and occurrences of psoriasis, a chronic skin disease.

In fact, many studies have shown that extreme stress can increase your susceptibility to virtually every major category of disease. For example, stress is one of the top risk factors for heart disease. A study from the *Journal of the American Medical Association* showed that negative emotions can even trigger a reduction in blood flow to the heart.

In my own medical practice, I've seen excessive stress worsen every possible hormone imbalance. Stress can exacerbate virtually every female problem, from PMS through post-menopause, by interfering with normal hormone production and function. I've seen this time and again in my practice. Women come in with severe PMS symptoms, fibroid tumors, and endometriosis, as well as hot flashes and insomnia. When I talk to them about what is going on in their personal life, more often than not, they tell me about an extremely stressful situation they are dealing with.

Unfortunately, even if you are eating the perfect diet, exercising every day, and taking the recommended nutritional supplements religiously, excessive stress can literally neutralize the benefits of everything positive that you are doing. But the good news is that the reverse is also true. You can create miracles by handling stress in a positive, self-nurturing, life-enhancing manner.

By discovering and taking the emotional and spiritual journey towards a stress-free life, you'll begin to notice several amazing changes. Your mood will lift and even out, you'll feel much more loving and joyful, you'll begin to sleep like a baby, you'll experience more positive dreams, and you'll have a new appreciation for your friends and family. What you may not also realize is that your health will greatly improve too, particularly your hormonal health.

Stress and Estrogen Deficiency

Like their estrogen dominant sisters, estrogen deficient-fast processors must also manage stress carefully. Not only can stress reduce estrogen levels, but it can reduce production of all sex hormones. This can lead to a worsening of menopausal symptoms, including hot flashes, insomnia, depression, and vaginal and tissue dryness, as well as other related issues, such as heart health.

A study from the journal *Menopause* looked at more than 400 women between the ages of 37 and 47 who were still menstruating. Researchers gave the participants an anxiety test at the start of the study and again six years later. By this time, many of the women were experiencing irregular periods and hot flashes.

The researchers found that those women with the highest anxiety levels had almost five times as many hot flashes as the less anxious women. Women with moderate anxiety had three times as many hot flashes. A second study from the *Maternal and Child Health Journal* found that vaginal dryness (also a common symptom of estrogen deficiency) was significantly associated with high emotional or psychological stress.

Lastly, a study from the *Annals of Internal Medicine* found that excessive stress was associated with increased risk of high blood pressure. Researchers found that stress reduction techniques such as deep breathing, biofeedback, meditation, yoga, and hypnosis all helped to reduce blood pressure.

Practice Deep Breathing and Meditation

One of the best things you can do for yourself is to discover the stress-reduction technique or techniques that are most beneficial to you. Regardless of your hormonal type, I've found that the foundation of any stress reduction program is to master the arts of deep breathing and meditation.

Next, I advocate using positive, life-affirming emotions to bring about renewed hormonal health. Specifically, we'll look at how prayer, love, gratitude, appreciation, laughter, happiness, optimism, positive self-image, forgiveness, and generosity can support and harmonize your health and hormones, relationships, job, and overall life and well-being.

I have taught deep breathing and meditation to patients. Without fail, they would tell me that they become much calmer, more patient, and happier after practicing these exercises. Best of all, a calm mind creates a calm body, and a calm body allows your autonomic nervous system to balance and slow down, your body chemistry to normalize, and your hormones to regain a much healthier state of balance.

To get ready for any stress reduction exercise, it's important that you take the following steps to prepare yourself:

1. Separate yourself physically and mentally from your normal, daily environment. Maybe designate a space in your home specifically for relaxation. It can include soothing pictures, a comfortable chair or couch, and possibly a sound machine.

2. Make sure you are wearing loose, comfortable clothing. Sit or lie down in a comfortable position. Try to make your spine as straight as possible and be sure to keep your arms and legs uncrossed.

3. Focus all of your attention on the stress reduction exercise you choose. Don't allow anything to distract you. Close your eyes and take a few deep, abdominal breaths. Focus on how the air goes in and out of your body.

These steps will help you separate your problems and concerns of the day from your relaxation practice so you can quiet your mind and begin to ease your mind, body, and soul.

General Relaxation Exercises

Regardless of their hormone status, the following exercises can benefit all women of any age. They include deep breathing, reducing muscle tension, and meditation.

Deep Breathing

Deep breathing is the foundation for any kind of stress relief. I have found that you must be able to control and be aware of your breathing if you want to relax your mind, body, or spirit. When you're physically or emotionally stressed, your breathing becomes more rapid and shallow. You may stop breathing altogether for brief periods without even realizing it. These changes in breathing patterns bring less life-sustaining oxygen into your lungs. At the same time, stress makes your muscles tense up, constricts your blood vessels to restrict blood flow, makes your heart beat faster, and stimulates the output of stressful chemicals from your adrenal glands.

All of these reactions decrease the amount of oxygen available to your cells, tissues, and organs. Poor oxygenation compromises a multitude of chemical reactions that are necessary for cell growth, maintenance, and repair. Energy production, waste removal, digestion, and other essential body processes are impaired. You feel fatigued, your body becomes less able to fight illness, and degenerative processes accelerate.

By breathing deeply, you are able to take in large amounts of oxygen. From your lungs, oxygen moves into your bloodstream where it binds to red blood cells and is transported to all the cells and tissues in your body. Oxygen helps your cells produce and utilize energy. When you exhale, waste products (carbon dioxide) are removed from your body through your lungs. This helps to optimize the oxygen levels throughout your body. Your muscles relax, your blood vessels dilate to increase blood flow, and your equilibrium returns, making you feel more energetic and balanced.

Similarly, your brain uses 20 percent of the oxygen in your body. If you don't get enough oxygen, mental clarity fades and you'll have barely enough energy to get by, and you'll lack your natural zest for life.

Next time you're stressed out—or feel stress coming on—try this deep abdominal breathing exercise:

1. Lie flat on your back with your knees pulled up. Keep your feet slightly apart. Try to breathe in and out through your nose.

2. Inhale deeply. As you breathe in, allow your stomach to relax so that the air flows into your abdomen. Your stomach should balloon out as you breathe in. Visualize your lungs filling with air as your chest swells out.

3. Imagine that the air you inhale is filling your body with energy.

4. Exhale deeply. As you breathe out, let your stomach and chest collapse. Imagine the air being pushed out, first from your abdomen and then from your lungs.

5. Imagine that the air you exhale is carrying away fatigue, concerns, and upset.

6. Repeat the process for three to five minutes, keeping your attention on your breath.

Reducing Muscle Tension

When stressed, most women store the tension in a certain group of muscles. Use this exercise to discover where the tension is, then how to release it from your body. This sequence is particularly important for women with emotional distress, such as anxiety and nervousness.

1. Lie on your back with your arms at your side, palms down.

2. Raise your right arm and keep it elevated for 15 seconds. Notice if your forearm feels tight and tense, or if the muscles are soft and pliable.

3. Let your arm drop back down to your side and relax. Your arm muscles should relax, too.

4. As you lie still, pay attention to other parts of your body that are tense, tight, or sore. Do any of your muscles have a dull ache?

5. Next, inhale deeply. As you breathe in, allow your stomach to relax so that the air flows into your abdomen. Let your stomach balloon out as you breathe in.

6. Imagine the breath is filled with love and relaxation. Let this positive energy travel and fill your muscles.

7. On your next exhalation, take the tension from your muscles and push them out of your body.

8. Continue this pattern of breathing in relaxation and breathing out tension until all of the tension in your muscles has melted away.

Meditation

Meditation allows you to create a state of deep relaxation, which is very healing to the entire body. Metabolism slows, as do physiological functions such as heart rate and blood pressure. Muscle tension decreases. Brain wave patterns shift from the fast beta waves that occur during a normal active day to the slower alpha waves that occur just before falling asleep, or in times of deep relaxation.

Try any or all of the following meditations.

Peace and Calm

1. Sit or lie in a comfortable position.

2. Close your eyes and breathe in and out deeply. Let your breathing be slow and relaxed.

3. Focus all of your attention on your breathing. Notice the movement of your chest and abdomen in and out.

4. Take yourself to a calm and peaceful place deep inside of you, and as you inhale, say the word "peace" to yourself. As you exhale, say the word "calm." Draw out the pronunciation of these words, so that they last for the entire breath.

5. Repeat this exercise for three to five minutes.

Breathing Meditation

1. Lie or sit in a very comfortable position.

2. Close your eyes and breathe deeply. Let your breathing be slow and relaxed.

3. Focus all of your attention on your breathing. Notice the movements of your chest and abdomen in and out.

4. Block out all other thoughts, feelings, and sensations. If you feel your attention wandering, bring it back to your breathing.

5. Say the word IN as you inhale. Say the word OUT as your exhale. Draw out the pronunciation of the word so that it lasts for the entire breath. The word IN sounds like this: i-i-i-i-n-n-n-n-n. The word OUT sounds like this: Ow-ow-w-w-w-w-t-t-t-t-t-t. Repeating these two words will help you to concentrate.

6. Do this exercise for as long as you are able to, up to several minutes.

Green Meadow

1. Lie on your back in a comfortable position. Inhale through your nose and exhale slowly and deeply through your mouth.

2. Visualize a beautiful green meadow full of lovely fragrant flowers. See yourself sitting or lying down on the grass In the middle of this meadow, feeling relaxed and calm. Feel the garden emanating peace and healing. You are the only person there in this still and peaceful place.

3. As you relax in this garden, you feel a healing energy fill every pore of your body with a warm, golden light. Every cell in your body that is in need of repair and healing is nourished by this light. This energy feels like a healing balm that relaxes you totally. All stress dissolves and fades from your mind. You feel totally at ease. Remain in this garden for as long as you wish.

4. When you are ready to leave, open your eyes and continue your slow, deep breathing for a few more cycles.

11

Exercise Supports Healthy Estrogen

Regular aerobic exercise is tremendously beneficial for women in menopause. Not only does it increase our level of energy, mental clarity, and balance our mood, but it also helps to maintain healthier estrogen and other hormone levels with our bodies.

Yet, the type of exercise that women who are suffering from menopause symptoms, like hot flashes, do is very important in terms of symptom reduction. For example, if you are suffering from hot flashes, you will aggravate your symptoms if you do hard, intense exercise and heat up your body and sweat. It is more important to maintain your yin reserves of fluid with slower, more expansive and relaxing aerobic activities that are moderately strenuous and can be done in a relaxed and leisurely way. Activities in this category include golf, swimming, walking, and bicycling at a leisurely pace. You can also try gardening and ballroom dancing, particularly the waltz. In other words, be more the "tortoise" than the "hare".

With these types of exercise, you will tend to breathe more deeply and slowly. Over time, this helps to improve the elasticity of your lungs and relaxes the diaphragm and chest muscles, thereby allowing you to inhale more oxygen. Moderate aerobic exercise also relaxes, dilates, and expands the network of blood vessels in the body, and enables the heart to work more efficiently. Better circulation and oxygenation improve the health of all your organs, including your ovaries and uterus.

Researchers Support Exercise's Medicinal Benefits

Exercise has been shown to benefit a whole host of health conditions, including menopausal symptoms, bone and heart health, libido, memory and cognitive function, and postmenopausal weight gain.

A study from the *Journal of Obstetrics and Gynecology* in Scandinavia found that just 21.5 percent of postmenopausal women who exercised regularly experienced hot flashes, as compared to 43.8 percent of women who lead a more sedentary life. Moreover, researchers discovered that those women who had no hot flashes at all exercised, on average, more than three hours a week. Those who exercised between two and three hours a week had moderate to severe hot flashes.

Another benefit of physical activity is the dilation (expansion) of the network of blood vessels so blood reaches the muscles and vital organs as well as the small capillaries. This can help reduce your risk for heart disease, as seen in a study from the *New England Journal of Medicine*. Researchers found that middle-aged and older women who walked just three hours per week cut their risk of heart disease by 30 to 40 percent.

I have also found that aerobic exercise, as well as a healthy diet, can enhance sexual desire and performance. Specifically, poor circulation can have a negative effect on libido and sexual performance. By increasing your level of aerobic activity, you are not only keeping your heart strong and healthy (a key concern for postmenopausal women) but you are ensuring a steady supply of blood flow to your entire pelvic region, including your vagina, which enhances sexual desire and vaginal lubrication.

Physical activity can improve mental alertness and cognitive function as well. It does this by opening up and dilating blood vessels of the head and brain, and by improving oxygenation and circulation to the brain and nerves. Thus, more nutrients can flow into this vital system, and more waste products can be removed.

An abundance of research shows that adults engaged in an active exercise program have better concentration, clearer thinking, and quicker problem-solving abilities. And a recent study in the *Journal of Internal Medicine* found that regular walking improved memory and reduced signs of dementia. The threshold for this positive effect was about 1,000 steps, or a little over a mile a day.

The *Journal of the American Medical Association* has also found that exercise helps women lose weight after menopause, thereby neutralizing the increase in breast cancer risk that accompanies even a small postmenopausal weight gain. This is supported by a study published in the *Journal of Gerontology*, which found that people between the ages of 60 and 70 who walked or jogged for 45 minutes several times a week for 9 to 12 months lost an average of 7 pounds, with the majority of the weight lost in the midsection. A positive association between reduction of abdominal fat and a decreased risk of heart disease and diabetes was also noted.

Several studies have shown that exercise is extremely helpful in easing osteoarthritis symptoms. According to research published in *The Gerontologist*, older patients with osteoarthritis in their lower extremities who engaged in an exercise program (flexibility, walking, and resistance training) for 2 to 12 months enjoyed statistically significant improvement in lower extremity stiffness and pain.

A similar study from the journal *Physical Therapy* divided 134 patients with osteoarthritis of the knee into two groups. Over the course of four weeks, the first group received supervised exercise, individualized manual therapy, and a home exercise program. The second group received the same home exercise program, as well as an office visit after two weeks. Researchers found that both groups had clinically and statistically significant improvement, with 52 percent improvement in the first group and 26 percent improvement in the second group.

Finally, exercise is extremely useful in relieving the symptoms of fibromyalgia. In fact, a study published in *Arthritis and Rheumatism* found that women with fibromyalgia who participated in a strength training and walking program for 20 weeks improved their muscle strength, endurance, and overall ability to function without aggravating their symptoms.

Building a Personal Exercise Program to Evaluate Your Fitness Level

As you move from a sedentary lifestyle to a regular exercise program, evaluate your level of fitness. It is important to know if you have any undiagnosed medical problems that could impact your proper level of activity. This includes problems such as thyroid disease, hypertension, and blood sugar imbalances commonly found in menopausal women. A complete medical examination is important for a menopausal woman beginning an exercise program after a long period of being sedentary.

Your physician should check your heart, lungs, pulse rate, and other physical parameters to evaluate your exercise fitness. In addition, blood and urine tests are frequently ordered. These tests can vary, based on the particular symptoms you report to your physician as well as the examination itself.

Depending on your age and symptoms, a general chemistry panel that checks the blood levels of minerals, as well as the health of various organs such as the thyroid, may a good idea. If you don't understand any terms or tests your physician uses, ask for more information. An informed and educated woman can do a much better job in planning and participating in her own wellness program. Once you have received a clean bill of health or understand any health limitations, you are ready to begin planning your exercise program.

Choosing an Exercise Program

No matter what type of exercise you choose to do, I recommend that you set aside 30 to 60 minutes each day to engage in regular aerobic exercise. If you've been sedentary, start with 10 minutes a day and work your way up to 30 minutes to an hour a day.

The type of exercise regimen you choose can vary greatly depending on the goals you wish to accomplish. If your main goal is to relieve menopause-related anxiety and stress and improve your general health and well-being, then aerobic exercise is best. This is because aerobic exercise promotes cardiovascular and respiratory health which, in turn, promotes relaxation and reduces the tendency toward menopause-related insomnia. Because it requires active work on the part of your skeletal and heart muscles, it reduces the muscle tension that often accompanies menopause-related nervous tension. Aerobic exercise includes jogging, walking, bicycle riding, skiing, swimming, dancing, jumping rope, and skating.

Women who are at high risk of osteoporosis will want to emphasize exercises that require weight-bearing stress on the long bones. Combining brisk walking with weight lifting or racquet sports can give the bones the workout they need and increase bone mass.

Women for whom sexuality is an important part of their emotional and physical well-being may find engaging in frequent sexual activity, or even massage, a pleasurable form of physical activity. For women who cannot participate in vigorous physical activity due to a pre-existing cardio-vascular condition (or lack of energy), then slower-paced activities such as golf or walking could provide a helpful degree of physical exercise as well as the benefits of socializing.

Many menopausal women notice the onset of arthritis symptoms or muscle tightness and tension during this time. As an antidote, I recommend exercises such as stretching that promote joint and muscle flexibility. Stretches are performed slowly, along with deep breathing, in a relaxed and careful manner. They are helpful in slowing down an anxious system whose physiology is set on overdrive.

Finally, gardening can promote peace of mind and relaxation along with physical activity. Pulling weeds and digging up the ground involve bending, lifting, and upper-body movements which rapidly dissipate anxiety.

Often, women may combine two or three types of exercise activities to meet a variety of goals. Whatever form of exercise you choose, make sure it meets the goals of promoting optimal health and well-being as well as providing abundant levels of energy.

Motivating Yourself to Exercise

If you encounter mental obstacles to beginning and sticking with a regular menopause exercise program, there are many ways to overcome this resistance. Be sure you are clear why you don't want to exercise so you can address the issues directly. Keeping the exercise diary found in the workbook section should help you pinpoint areas of resistance.

- Exercise at the time of day that feels most natural. For example, if you are a late riser, don't try to exercise early in the morning. Exercise when you are the least hurried and stressed by your schedule. If your longest amount of free time is in the late afternoon between work and dinner, put aside that time to engage in physical activity.

- Exercise in an attractive setting. If you run or walk, pick a setting near you that promotes peace and calm. Walk or run in a park, on a beach, or on a quiet residential street. Avoid areas with lots of cars and traffic congestion. Exercise with a friend or support person. This can be a great help in motivating and encouraging you to begin and stick with an exercise program.

- Use your mind to disconnect from your daily activities. Positive mental exercises can help you relax before starting physical activity. Many women find that a few minutes of doing visualizations (seeing themselves performing and enjoying the exercise routine in their minds) or saying affirmations (making positive statements about the benefits of exercise) prepares them for their exercise routine.

- Listen to music while you exercise. Many women find that the exercise period goes by more quickly and the process is more fun and enjoyable while listening to music. Be sure to choose.

- Be sure to choose an exercise activity that you enjoy. Don't pick an activity that you find boring. Refer to the activity chart at the end of this chapter if you need help in selecting an activity that looks interesting.

Beginning an Exercise Program for Menopause

Before you begin a menopause-relief exercise program, read the following guidelines. They will help you perform your exercise in an optimally beneficial manner. These guidelines are particularly useful for women just beginning regular exercise after leading a sedentary lifestyle. Getting a good start when beginning the program can make a major difference in how well you enjoy and stick to your chosen physical activity.

- During the first week or two of your program, build up your exercise level gradually. Keep initial exercise workouts short. Increase the length of your sessions by five-minute increments until you are exercising between 30 and 60 minutes per session.

- Exercise in a relaxed and unhurried manner. Set aside adequate time so you do not feel rushed. Anytime you feel anxiety, panic, or excessive muscle tension, stop the exercise. Then, re-evaluate your pace to see if it is too vigorous. Initially you might want to exercise with another person who can provide support and companionship.

- Wear loose, comfortable clothing. If you are doing stretch work without socks to give your feet complete freedom of movement and to prevent slipping.

- Evacuate your bowels and/or bladder before you begin to exercise. Try to exercise at least 90 minutes before a meal and wait at least 2 hours after eating to exercise. Working out before dinner is particularly good because it helps diffuse tension that has accumulated throughout the day.

- Avoid exercising when ill or extremely stressed. Instead, do the stress-reduction exercises provided in this book.

- Move slowly and carefully when starting each exercise session. This promotes muscle flexibility and helps prevent injury

- Breathe deeply and evenly when you are exercising; this will give you more endurance and you will tire less easily.

- Always rest for a few minutes after completing the exercises.

Activities for Menopausal Women
- walking
- bicycle riding
- skiing
- swimming
- aerobic dancing
- low-impact aerobics
- ice skating
- roller skating
- tennis
- ping-pong
- golf
- croquet
- bowling
- stretching
- weight lifting
- gardening

Benefits of Exercise
- Helps relieve hot flashes
- Helps relieve vaginal and bladder atrophy
- Relieves anxiety, irritability, insomnia and depression
- Helps prevent osteoporosis
- Conditions the heart, lungs, and muscles
- Helps prevent heart disease
- Helps control weight and improve appearance
- Improves function of vital organs such as digestive tract and nervous system
- Improves strength, stamina and flexibility
- Increases vigor and energy

About Susan M. Lark, M.D.

Dr. Susan Lark is one of the foremost authorities in the fields of women's health care and alternative medicine. Dr. Lark has successfully treated many thousands of women emphasizing holistic health and complementary medicine in her clinical practice. Her mission is to provide women with unique, safe and effective alternative therapies to greatly enhance their health and well-being.

A graduate of Northwestern University Feinberg School of Medicine, she has served on the clinical faculty of Stanford University Medical School, and taught in their Division of Family and Community Medicine.

Dr. Lark is a distinguished clinician, author, lecturer and innovative product developer. Through her extensive clinical experience, she has been an innovator in the use of self-care treatments such as diet, nutrition, exercise and stress management techniques in the field of women's health, and has lectured extensively throughout the United States on topics in preventive medicine. She is the author of many best-selling books on women's health. Her signature line of nutritional supplements and skin care products are available through healthydirections.com.

One of the most widely referenced physicians on the Internet, Dr. Lark has appeared on numerous radio and television shows, and has been featured in magazines and newspapers including: Real Simple, Reader's Digest, McCall's, Better Homes & Gardens, New Woman, Mademoiselle, Harper's Bazaar, Redbook, Family Circle, Seventeen, Shape, Great Life, The New York Times, The Chicago Tribune, and The San Francisco Chronicle.

She has also served as a consultant to major corporations, including the Kellogg Company and Weider Nutrition International, and was spokesperson for The Gillette Company Women's Cancer Connection.

Dr. Lark can be contacted at (650) 561-9978 to make an appointment for a consultation.

We would enjoy hearing from you! Please share your success stories, requests for new topics and comments with us. Our team at Womens Wellness Publishing may be contacted at yourstory@wwpublishing.com. We invite you to visit our website for Dr. Lark's newest books at womenswellnesspublishing.com.

Dr. Susan's Solutions
Health Library For Women

The following books are available from Amazon.com, Amazon Kindle, iTunes, Womens Wellness Publishing and other major booksellers. Dr. Susan is frequently adding new books to her health library.

Women's Health Issues

Dr. Susan's Solutions: Healthy Heart and Blood Pressure
Dr. Susan's Solutions: Healthy Menopause
Dr. Susan's Solutions: The Anemia Cure
Dr. Susan's Solutions: The Bladder Infection Cure
Dr. Susan's Solutions: The Candida-Yeast Infection Cure
Dr. Susan's Solutions: The Chronic Fatigue Cure
Dr. Susan's Solutions: The Cold and Flu Cure
Dr. Susan's Solutions: The Endometriosis Cure
Dr. Susan's Solutions: The Fibroid Tumor Cure
Dr. Susan's Solutions: The Irregular Menstruation Cure
Dr. Susan's Solutions: The Menstrual Cramp Cure
Dr. Susan's Solutions: The PMS Cure

Emotional and Spiritual Balance

Breathing Meditations for Healing, Peace and Joy
Dr. Susan's Solutions: The Anxiety and Stress Cure

Women's Hormones

DHEA: The Fountain of Youth Hormone
Healthy, Natural Estrogens for Menopause
Pregnenolone: Your #1 Sex Hormone
Progesterone: The Superstar of Hormone Balance
Testosterone: The Hormone for Strong Bones, Sex Drive and Healthy Menopause

Diet and Nutrition

Dr. Susan Lark's Healing Herbs for Women
Dr. Susan Lark's Complete Guide to Detoxification
Enzymes: The Missing Link to Health
Healthy Diet and Nutrition for Women: The Complete Guide
Renew Yourself Through Juice Fasting and Detoxification Diets

Energy Therapies and Anti-Aging

Acupressure for Women: Relieve Symptoms of Dozens of Health Issues Through Pressure Points

Exercise and Flexibility

Stretching and Flexibility for Women
Stretching Programs for Women's Health Issues

About Womens Wellness Publishing

"Bringing Radiant Health and Wellness to Women"

Womens Wellness Publishing was founded to make a positive difference in the lives of women and their families. We are the premier publisher of print and eBooks focused on women's health and wellness. We are committed to publishing the finest quality and most comprehensive line of books that covers every area that a woman needs to create vibrant health and a joyful, fulfilling life.

Our books are written and created by the top health and wellness experts who share with you, our readers, their wisdom and extensive experience successfully treating many thousands of patients.

We encourage you to browse through our online bookstore; new books are frequently being added at womenswellnesspublishing.com. Also visit our Lifestyle Center and Customer Bonus Center for more exciting and helpful health and wellness information and resources.

Follow us on Facebook for the latest health tips, recipes, and all natural solutions to many women's health issues (facebook.com/wwpublishing).

About Our Associate Program

We invite you to become part of the Womens Wellness Publishing Community through our Associate Program. You will have the opportunity to earn generous commissions on sales that you create through your blog, social network, support groups, community groups, school & alumni groups, friends, family or other networks.

To join our program, go to our website and click "Become an Associate" (womenswellnesspublishing.com). We support your sales and marketing efforts by offering you and your customers:

- Free support materials with updates on all of our new book releases, promotions, and bonuses for you and your customers
- Free audio downloads, booklets, and guides
- Special discounts and sales promotions

Made in the USA
San Bernardino, CA
19 March 2014